Contents

Foreword

Leadership and learning are indispensable to each other.
(John F Kennedy, speech prepared for delivery on
the day of his assassination.)

If we are to work in effective teams and deliver effective healthcare then leadership is vital. This book encourages us to apply what we learn about leadership to our teams, whether we are in general medical, dental or ophthalmic practice; yet is readily applicable to leadership in many walks of life. It is also readily applicable at various levels within teams. Leadership is about much more than being in charge, and is a vital element of professional practice; yet in my experience it is barely mentioned in undergraduate studies or in postgraduate programmes. Along with many others I have had the good fortune to participate in the excellent leadership programmes that have sprung up over recent years. But participating in such a programme one quickly realises that leaders are always learning and, I hope, always aspiring to become good enough leaders. Often I find myself reflecting on events and wishing that I had handled them better. Which of us with any degree of insight can honestly say otherwise? Look at your own environment and honestly evaluate the qualities of the leadership and of team-work. Each of us can learn more and this book is an excellent foundation for this learning. Clare Mullins and Graham Constable provide a tangible and practical resource drawing on their wealth of experience of business and the NHS, and of general practice in particular. They demonstrate a clear understanding of our world that is firmly grounded in insightful experience.

Leadership is about more than management and it is not necessarily the same as being in charge. As the authors say, managers need to exhibit leadership but leaders should not necessarily be performing management tasks.

This book is incredibly well referenced. If you have heard any management guru spouting forth jargon or spent any time looking at the business section in airport bookshops you will recognise the references, but the difference herein is that they are clearly and practically explained and put to practical use. This is not some simple self-help guide; it is a practical, thorough and useful text. It starts by recognising that leadership, learning and team building all take time and helps to release that time. It then perceptively explores aspects of leadership with chapters having suggested learning outcomes and action points, practical examples and space to encourage reflection and application. But its greatest strength is to realise that leaders need teams to lead and teams need leaders. The later focus on team building ensures that our learning is readily applied.

Once you have read, reflected and applied your learning about leadership and teams I challenge you to look at quality of healthcare and quality improvement from a leadership stand point and from a team perspective. Not only do our teams need leadership but our patients deserve it. I commend the authors and this book to you and commend the concept of applying leadership to teambuilding.

Dr Simon Gregory FRCGP MMEd ILTM
Dean of Postgraduate General Practice Education
East Midlands Healthcare Workforce Deanery
Leicester UK
December 2006

About the authors

Clare Mullins has been a physiotherapist for 12 years working in hospitals, general practices and her own business in Australia and England. She discovered early in her career that she was equally fascinated with how people's minds *and* bodies worked which led her to become a qualified life coach. Since then she has formed Growing Professionals and offers coaching and training to make working lives easier in the medical world. She does this by developing people's skills in leadership and communication, as well as building their confidence to implement those skills.

Graham Constable was a commissioned officer in the Royal Air Force following which he co-founded a professional services company. He has 20 years of business experience nationally and internationally encompassing operations, business development, change management, organisational growth and value management. He is a partner in Growing Professionals and the founder of The Business Tree. He works with executives and managers bringing about change, breakthrough development and growth of individuals, groups and teams. He garners the innate experience, knowledge and expertise of people within organisations to cultivate great teams.

Introduction

'We know we have a dysfunctional nursing team but we're ignoring it because it doesn't affect the rest of the surgery.'

'I don't want to just tell people what to do, but the consultation approach doesn't seem to get anything done. What else can I do?'

'There's a feeling of ''us'' and ''them'' between the doctors and the admin team but that's the same everywhere, isn't it?'

'I want to know what my leadership style is.'

These are the kinds of phrases we frequently heard when talking to clinicians and practice managers in primary care. There were lots of statements about dysfunctional relationships, problems between entire teams, the negative impact of constant change, the challenges of handling difficult behaviour by staff and how difficult it was to lead when they had little or no training in this area.

What was more concerning were the common approaches to such problems, i.e. the 'if we ignore it, it might go away' approach or 'I'll figure it out as I go along'. But, like a crack in a dam wall, these problems never went away. They only got worse and eventually the dam wall burst. And if they were learning as they 'went along' then it was often a long, difficult and unfulfilling path.

Ultimately there were common themes within these problems which boiled down to a lack of leadership and teamwork. Most often this was not from lack of trying. The people we spoke to were sometimes at their wits' end and feeling like failures having tried so many things so many times. Sometimes they knew what they could be doing but lacked the confidence to put it into action and other times they just didn't have enough tools to handle the situation.

In searching for resources to address these problems we found year-long courses, one-hour seminars and books that provided a lot of theory but left the question 'So how do I actually do that?'. So we decided to fill the gap by writing this book. We have aimed to produce an easy-to-use, 'how to' guide to enable you to develop your leadership and teambuilding skills in the context of your work in primary care. Throughout the book there are practical exercises for you to complete and at the end of each chapter you will find suggested learning outcomes and action points to help you focus.

The purpose of this book is to equip you with the skills, tools and attitudes necessary to become better leaders and to develop individuals and teams around you. You will find practical advice to help you in your day-to-day role. Because we want you to actually *do* something different, there is a strong coaching and personal development slant to this book rather than a recital of theories. As a result there are a lot of exercises you may choose to do.

As with any new skills, how much you gain from this book will depend on how much you actually *do*. Reading this, but not changing any of your thoughts, actions or behaviours, will mean no practical change in your workplace at all. So we encourage you to take this saying to heart:

> *If you always do what you always did, then you'll always get what you always got.*

We also don't expect this book to be the complete answer for all of you. It aims to provide a good foundation for you to explore and develop further from. We encourage you to seek out mentors, coaches, seminars, courses and programmes to stimulate your development in these areas and help you implement it all. Some of the information here may seem like a statement of the obvious, but even though this is the case, it is neither obvious nor easy to put into action.

Before starting we want to address a couple of common debates.

Nature versus nurture

We believe that some people fit into leadership roles more comfortably than others; however, leadership capability which involves behaviours, attitudes and skills *can be learned by anyone*.

Leadership versus management

Leadership is generally seen as the job of those who either own or run a business including general practices and hospitals. It's what those people at the 'top' are meant to do.

Leaders address the big picture. They determine vision and direction of a business, the strategy or plan to get there, engaging their staff to support and pursue that vision and monitoring progress. By comparison, managers tend to the detail, creating systems for efficient business operations, maximising the performance of individuals and teams, developing service and business innovations and problem solving as needed.

There is clearly an overlap here in the area of people handling which we believe is the area that requires the strongest leadership capability. So managers need to exhibit leadership too. Leaders however should not be performing 'management' tasks, at least not on a regular basis. It is a sign of an ineffective leader if they are involved in the minutiae of projects or daily operations. This shows that they have either recruited the wrong people to management level, not developed their managers to do their jobs to a high enough standard or have not addressed their own difficulty with delegating and trusting others to do their job.

What you will find in this book

Based on feedback from clients, we've started the book with a time-management chapter. They described how valuable the leadership and teambuilding information was, but they hadn't really applied it in the workplace because other more urgent things had taken priority. So we encourage you to find time in your schedule to put what you read into action.

We then cover:

- a leadership model applicable to any situation that requires a task to be achieved
- leadership styles to use in different situations and with different people as well as the skills and attitudes you need to bring each style to life
- a five-step process to become a better leader
- fundamental information about teams
- how to assess teams and maximise their performance
- a process to fix dysfunctional teams
- the essential supports that will make it easier for you to bring your leadership and team-development skills to life
- difficult situations that require 'extra-strength' leadership.

Lastly we have used words that you may normally associate with the business, not the medical, world. Our experience is that sometimes people resist 'management speak' and the concept of healthcare as a business because they associate it with overcharging and underserving their customers. This is not what we want for your business. Instead, we'd like you to think of your business as being the best provider of the best service and the best place to work.

We hope that you enjoy this book and reap the rewards that come from being a strong leader and team builder.

With warmest regards,
Clare and Graham

Chapter 1

The case for leadership and strong teams

Why bother with leadership skills?

Imagine you are a patient attending your local general practice for the first time. You enter the reception area and queue behind three other people. You cannot help but overhear the conversation between the receptionist and the elderly gentleman at the head of the queue trying to make an appointment. You can hear the frustration in the receptionist's voice. There are two more receptionists nearby but they are doing paperwork, chatting to each other and avoiding looking in your direction.

Eventually, the gentleman is given an appointment and begins to leave but looks anxious and a little confused. The receptionist glances at her colleagues with a look of irritation and turns to the next person in line with a heavy sigh, asking 'Yes?'.

You wait while the other people are attended to and then are told to 'take a seat in the waiting area'. While you look for a sign or direction to the waiting room one of the doctors appears. Her request for one of the receptionists to find the test results for a patient is met with a sigh. Once the doctor leaves, the receptionist complains, quite audibly, to her colleague about the expectations of doctors for them to drop everything when they want something done.

You still don't know where you are going so ask another stony-faced receptionist and are pointed upstairs. Twenty minutes past your appointment time, the doctor you saw earlier appears and calls your name. She apologises for being late and asks how she can help as you sit down. As you tell her of the medication that you need for your migraines, she scans the computer screen for your registration details and history. Your prescriptions are produced and you are told to collect them at the dispensary downstairs. You mention that you are looking for lifestyle advice on how to better manage your migraines but she apologises and tells you to make another appointment as she doesn't have time to deal with that today. You leave wondering if the doctor will have time at your next appointment and how receptionists in a customer-facing position can be so miserable and get away with it.

By the end of the day, the doctor finishes her clinic an hour late and decides to come in early the next day to do admin tasks. As she drives home she tries to put work to the back of her mind. She doesn't want her angst to affect her husband and young daughter but it's getting harder to leave work at work. The grumpy receptionists, the volume of patients, the enormous amount of administration tasks . . . the list goes on and she wonders: 'Is running a business worth all this hassle?'

Does any of this sound familiar? The staff that won't help each other, the rudeness to patients and colleagues, the stressed doctor running late who struggles to run a business, do their job and maintain a normal family life?

Your situation might not be this extreme but these are the results of a workplace without leadership or a sense of collaboration and the costs are enormous. In this fictional workplace the owners can soon expect patient complaints, loss of patients to other practices, staff absenteeism from being run down or apathetic, resignations from their good workers, lower levels of patient care, lower income and difficulty recruiting good staff. Add to this the low morale and lack of joy that comes from working in such an environment and the consequent reduction in productivity. The doctors are also so busy seeing patients and just existing day to day that they can't be involved in developing their business or taking advantage of new developments in their profession. This means that they may miss the chance for their business to become more profitable, to offer additional services for patients or provide more benefits to staff.

The end result is a failing or at least a struggling business.

So what's the solution?

The solution lies in the people and in those who lead them.

People are the foundation on which all service industry businesses are built. You match the right people to the right jobs and let them work according to their strengths. You inspire them to look to the future, create challenging goals and be creative in how those goals are achieved. You encourage reasonable risk and mistakes in the spirit of learning and development. You give them responsibilities, keep them on track and reward them. You create with them the standards and procedures that make the business perform and you ensure that they operate according to those standards and procedures. You inspire loyalty and trust, you demand accountability and encourage involvement from everyone.

Once you have this, the results naturally follow.

To get the most from your people and to implement and sustain these things, there must be strong leadership and a strong sense of being part of an important team. Most of this comes down to understanding how people think and behave. There are of course other skills involved in being a great leader but unless you have a good understanding of how people tick, particularly in their workplace, you will struggle as a leader.

Before you begin the process of becoming a better leader, consider this sample of studies on people behaviour and bear the results in mind as you work through this book and reflect on what's happening in your workplace today.

Frederick Herzberg[1] studied what motivated people in the late 1950s and went on to form his theory that there are two dimensions to job satisfaction. He found that what made people dissatisfied were 'hygiene' issues, which included company policies, supervision, salary, interpersonal relations, working conditions, status and security. If these were absent or inappropriate, employees felt dissatisfied. However, in order to feel satisfied, employees needed the 'intrinsic motivators', which included achievement, recognition, work itself, responsibility, advance-ment and growth. Importantly, the hygiene areas had to be addressed first to allow the motivators to have an effect.

This means: There are certain factors that cause motivation and others that cause lack of motivation. If an employer wants their staff to feel satisfied and motivated at work they must meet the hygiene factors first and then provide intrinsic motivators.

Elton Mayo's[2] famous Hawthorne experiments from 1924 to 1933 demonstrated that the productivity of factory workers rose when Mayo made changes to the workplace. These included the number and length of breaks they had, the amount of light they worked with and changing their work hours. What was most interesting was that no matter what the change, productivity increased. In one experiment Mayo saw an increase in productivity when the lights were 'turned up' and it rose even higher when he turned them down again. In another experiment, he added extra breaks, a hot meal and fewer hours of work to a team of women resulting in greater productivity and saw a further increase in productivity when he took those things away again.

This means: The various experiments demonstrated that showing an interest in staff, engaging them in business development, asking them for help and nurturing a sense of community yielded greater commitment and productivity.

Robert Rosenthal[3] of Harvard University showed that groups of children taught by teachers who thought they were not as clever as other groups of children consistently underperformed in exams. So the expectations of the teacher determined their performance and a self-fulfilling prophecy occurred. This effect has since been reproduced in the business world, particularly by Alfred Oberlander in the 1960s.[4] His organisational experiments showed raised productivity and morale in the groups that were requested to deliver particularly high results.

This means: Your expectations of people, be they good or bad, will usually come true.

Berlew and Hall[5] performed a study of college graduates working in their first year as managers at AT&T and found that both expectations and performance in the first year correlated consistently with later performance and success. They concluded that 'meeting high company expectations in the critical first year leads to the internalisation of positive job attitudes and high standards'.

This means: The first year that a new employee is with you is the most vital for ingraining in them the standards and expectations of the business or department and for supporting them to succeed.

W Chan Kim and Renee Mauborgne[6] researched the links between trust, idea sharing and corporate performance in the 1990s. They showed a direct link between using a 'fair process' and employees' attitudes of trust and commitment, behaviour of voluntary cooperation and performance levels that exceeded expectations. Importantly they noted that fair process 'is not decision by consensus. It does not set out to achieve harmony or to win people's support through compromises'.

This means: Using a fair process for disciplinary matters results in positive outcomes in attitudes, behaviour and performance among staff. So don't be afraid to discipline people and hold them accountable to standards. Just be sure that all the staff know and understand the fair process that you use.

The case for being a great leader and teambuilder in your practice shows clear benefits for those leading, for the staff and customers including the patients and other organisations that you work with. There is a lot to understand and do in order to become a better leader. The first place to start therefore is finding the time to put into practice what you are about to read.

References

1 Herzberg F. How do you motivate employees? *Harvard Business Review.* 2003; **81**(1): 86–96.
2 Mayo E. Cited in: Nicholson N. How to motivate your problem people. *Harvard Business Review.* 2003; **81**(1): 57–65.
3 Rosenthal R. Cited in: Sterling Livingston J. Pygmalion in management. *Harvard Business Review.* 2003; **81**(1): 97–106.
4 Oberlander A. Cited in: Sterling Livingston J. Pygmalion in management. *Harvard Business Review.* 2003; **81**(1): 97–106.
5 Berlew DE, Hall DT. Cited in: Sterling Livingston J. Promotion in management. *Harvard Business Review.* 2003; **81**(1): 97–106.
6 Chan Kim W, Mauborgne R. Fair process: managing in the knowledge economy. *Harvard Business Review.* 2004; **81**(1): 127–136.

Chapter 2

Finding time

Managing yourself, other people and the workplace (YOW)

First of all, there is no such thing as 'time management'. That would mean you could change the length of day and night! However, you can manage yourself, other people and your environment. You can also prioritise and categorise activities so you know what you need to invest the most time in and when. This brings us to the 'YOW' question which is 'What role are You, Other people and the Workplace playing in creating or exacerbating time-related issues?'.

Consider the last time you thought 'this is such a waste of time'. What were you doing? Were you trying to find a form in a cluttered office, were you mumbling to yourself as someone talked your ear off or were you thinking 'I wish I hadn't agreed to do this'? Each of these scenarios can be improved by using the following process either with your team or on a one-to-one basis.

The process

First, establish useful **ground rules** for this whole process such as being objective, open, honest, solution focused and having a 'no-blame' approach. The best way to do this is ask the group what they could do to make this process a complete failure, and what they could do to make it a complete success. Once you have this list, which actually are behaviours, request them to agree to embrace the 'success' behaviours and not the 'failure' behaviours. This will keep participants on track and if you need to correct anyone's behaviour, you are noting a move away from a standard they have agreed to, rather than making a personal attack.

Second, **brainstorm** with your team the activities in the practice that either waste or use time inefficiently. Make a long list, then agree and prioritise the issues that if improved would have the greatest positive impact.

Now ask the YOW question in relation to each of the prioritised issues in order to establish root causes of these problems. The most difficult part of this exercise is for people to acknowledge how they are contributing to the problem. Begin with the Other people and Workplace areas, then encourage them to explore their role individually. Offering suggestions can help to get people thinking as most haven't done this kind of self-exploration.

Managing you

Key questions:

- What is happening *in you* when you are struggling to meet time frames or feel your time is being wasted?
- Are you avoiding admitting there is just too much work for you to handle?

- Are you avoiding hurting someone's feelings?
- How do you feel if you have to challenge another person?
- How often do you feel you are picking up the pieces of someone's errors?
- How often do you feel you are the only person who can do the job properly?
- Do you think it is your job to solve all the problems?

Get people to report to the group what they are comfortable with sharing. As the leader, go first – to demonstrate what you want them to consider and also to show that you are human and make mistakes too.

An open discussion can then follow about each other's concerns. For example:

- Someone who thinks they are the only one who can do the job properly, but is stressed because they are so busy, can take the opportunity to find out who is best suited to be trained or coached so they can delegate extra work.
- Someone who worries about upsetting a particular colleague can check whether they really would be upsetting them if they were to say no to extra work or if their colleague will happily wait or delegate the work elsewhere.

Naturally you can't force people to talk openly about these potentially sensitive issues, so give them the option of seeing you privately. If common issues arise then arrange a training event specific to the needs of the group (e.g. assertiveness).

Managing others

This area is **not** about blaming others for difficult situations and absolving yourself. This is about finding the most effective way to relate and communicate with others and about accepting that what works for you may not necessarily work for them.

For example: I coached a doctor who admitted feeling really stressed and irritated by a particular receptionist in his practice. He felt that she wasted his time when she came to give him messages. It had reached the stage that she only had to appear in his doorway for his mood to drop. The problem that he had was the way she communicated with him. She would give him every detail, and more, about a question or problem that needed solving, while he just wanted her to get to the point. She talked in essays; he talked in bullet points.

The solution involved him first recognising their different styles and second requesting her to speak to him in bullet points. He explained to her that for him to be most effective in hearing and responding to her, she needed to give him a summary only and if he needed further information he would definitely come to her for that. She felt confident that he was hearing her and he was much happier with their communications. It was a win-win situation.

Where there are issues like this, have a conversation with the express purpose of improving communication between both parties. Start by asking how they would prefer you to communicate with them. Then it's your turn.

- Do they prefer to talk in bullet points or essays?
- Do they prefer to write requests down so they don't forget them?
- Are they happy with verbal instructions?

In the example above, the doctor also had to change the way he spoke to the receptionist, giving her more detail than he normally would and checking with her: 'Have I given you enough information? Are you happy with that?'

Another vital element in managing other people involves the essential leadership skill of enabling your colleagues and staff through coaching, training, supporting and trust. If you have a problem with delegating because the staff don't have the necessary skills, then you will need to start training and supporting someone who has the potential and enthusiasm for the jobs that need delegating. This is covered in Chapters 8 and 9. Alternatively, if there are skills that can be learned through an external provider, it may be cheaper to send the person on a course.

Managing the workplace

This means considering how your physical environment, equipment and operating procedures are helping and/or hindering you in your goal of being more effective. This is covered in detail in Chapter 10 (from p. 93). Suffice to say your physical environment affects your energy levels, information transfer, learning and relationships and your equipment and operating procedures affect your efficiency.

A crucial element in freeing time for you to lead and build your teams is operating procedures. When you look at how your week or month is structured, where do you have protected or planning time? If you don't have any, you may need to commit some of your personal time to learning and to creating action.

An example of managing all YOW elements

A doctor described to me how she would frequently have her time wasted by the support staff in her general practice. She told how her door would be open and people would lean against the door frame and start chatting. She was usually working on the computer trying to catch up on patient notes. Her usual approach was to keep looking at the computer in a half-hearted attempt to keep working but she would also acknowledge the other person's conversation with 'It's OK, keep talking'. Surprise surprise! The person was in no hurry to leave.

When she applied the YOW question to this situation she identified that she was giving the message that she was happy for the person to chat, even though she wanted them to leave. She also identified that she did this because she didn't want to cause offence. Additionally, the workplace component of having her door open was also perceived as an invitation to chat. The other person who initially seemed to be the source of the problem turned out to have a very minor role.

The solution to her time-wasting situation was to manage herself and her environment. She started closing the door when she needed to focus and she found words that she was comfortable with to tell people she couldn't chat at that moment and needed to work.

Prioritising and categorising

There are two methods that I recommend to people for categorising and prioritising their activities.

Table 2.1 Time Management Matrix. (Source: Covey.[1])

Quadrant I *Urgent–important activities* Crises such as patient illness, inappropriate or aggressive behaviour, computer system failure. Deadline-driven projects such as qualities and outcomes framework submission.	*Quadrant II* *Not urgent–important activities* Team and relationship building. Strategic and tactical planning. Management tasks. Performance appraisals. Staff meetings.
Quadrant III *Urgent–not important activities* Most interruptions. Some phone calls, meetings, emails and reports.	*Quadrant IV* *Not urgent–not important activities* Some mail, emails and phone calls. Superficial chatting.

1 **Stephen Covey's Time Management Matrix**[1] classifies activities as being important or not important and urgent or not urgent (*see* Table 2.1).

Whether something is 'urgent' or not is related to time. If it is urgent, it requires immediate attention.

Whether something is 'important' or not has to do with the results or outcome of doing that action. If it is important then investing time in it will have a positive outcome.

Some examples:

Urgent–important

- If someone collapses and stops breathing, this is an urgent–important situation. The consequences are important and will depend on the time taken to administer care.
- Submitting people's time sheets becomes urgent if they have been left to the last minute as people's mortgage payments are important.

Important–not urgent

- Planning the strategy to achieve your vision is important. It's not urgent however as there is no set time frame to achieve it by.
- Teambuilding and development exercises for individual teams and the practice team.
- Updates on progress toward goals such as reducing waiting times for patients.

Urgent–not important

- 'Emergency' appointments in general practice taken by people without a serious medical condition.
- Some interruptions by staff, such as a nurse asking about a patient even though if the question isn't answered immediately it won't affect the patient's health.

Not important–not urgent

- Chit-chat when you are avoiding work.
- Personal phone calls or emails.

If most of your activities fit in quadrants I and III then you will probably feel that you are being controlled by situations and other people. This is a recipe for feeling very stressed.

If you are in quadrant II then you will be working on tasks that produce important results, have a more rewarding experience and as a result you will spend less time in quadrants I or III.

If you are in quadrant IV, you will probably be disciplined or fired soon.

Use this categorising system to evaluate your activities and *invest as much time as possible in quadrant II* and your remaining time in quadrant I.

2   **The Time-Usage Continuum** allows you to classify your activities on a scale from being a 'waste' of time to being an 'investment'.

Waste	Neutral	Investment

A waste of time means that you get no reward from that activity – for example, looking for paperwork that you have 'lost'.

An investment of time gives you a return or reward – for example, developing a deeper relationship with your colleagues or taking further studies.

A neutral activity is something that doesn't give you a reward but is not a waste of time either.

These categories are subjective and what is a neutral activity to one person may not be to another. It's important to recognise that although you may feel something is a waste of time, look at it objectively to see if there actually is a positive outcome. Chatting with staff about personal lives may feel like a waste but may result in greater trust in the relationship.

Use the language in this categorising system as a trigger for you to take action. Next time you are thinking 'this is a waste of time', do something about it.

Time waster to time investor

Where does time go?

A lot of my clients have become so busy that they don't know where their time goes in a day. Keeping a 'Daily Activity Diary' helps to give you a baseline on the activities you do and don't do in any given day or week. A copy can be downloaded from www.claremullins.com/resources.html.

Exercise: What you do with your time

To use the Daily Activity Diary, record every 10 minutes the activity you are doing. If interruptions come up, note who is involved and what the interruption is about. You need to keep the diary for at least one week which reflects an 'average' week for you. This is an intensive exercise but a valuable one. Often, changing some of the little things that waste time makes an enormous difference to your total time available in a day or week.

When you review your diary, look for patterns of activity in relation to times of day, people involved and days of the week. For example, you may find that Monday mornings are full of interruptions. Ask the YOW question ('What role are You, Other people and the Workplace playing in this example?') to discover the underlying reasons for this and then explore strategies to reduce your interruptions. If, however, the interruptions are necessary then this is the time to do tasks that require short periods of attention.

Also look for what's missing such as lunch breaks, time for exercise or relaxation, time with family and friends, and hours of sleep. Consider what is really important to you and then see how much time you invest in those activities.

Exercise: In an ideal world!

Now describe your 'ideal working week' and your 'ideal year' that shows what you are moving toward.

Imagine you are ordering from a restaurant menu and I'm here to take your order.

- What time would you like to start work?
- What time would you like to finish?
- How long for a lunch break? And what time would you like that?
- Any coffee breaks? And how long would you like those to be?
- How much face-to-face clinical time do you want? And how much non-face-to-face clinical time will you need to support that?
- What else would you like to take time for? Committee involvement, research . . .?
- How many holidays would you like each year? Any study sabbaticals?
- Any long weekends or regular days off?

Think in more detail about what you want to achieve in your workplace and home life and write a list of what you need to do to achieve that. For example, at work if you are aiming to develop your team then regular meetings will be necessary. How much time do you need to allocate for those meetings?

What from your list can you realistically start doing now? Use the Weekly Activity Diary (available at www.claremullins.com/resources.html) to record your ideal week and your current week, so you have a goal to work toward.

Exercise: Inspiration

The purpose of writing your ideal week is to give you the inspiration to start doing things differently. So imagine yourself working your ideal week. How do you feel? How do you look? What are your patients saying to you? What is your family saying? What are your friends noticing?

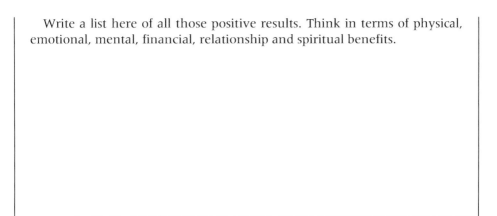

Write a list here of all those positive results. Think in terms of physical, emotional, mental, financial, relationship and spiritual benefits.

What's stopping you?

The most common obstacle for people wanting to change the way they work is difficulty saying 'no'.

How to say 'no'

Are you the kind of person who is virtually programmed to say 'yes' as soon as you are asked to do something? Your brain registers a request, your mouth opens, the word flies out and suddenly you've agreed to something you don't really want to do or you have become seriously overcommitted. 'Yes' is your default response. And usually this is followed by 'Of course, it's no trouble at all' as you quietly think 'What the hell am I saying?!'. Well, you are not alone!

Why we say 'yes' and what to do about it

1   Habit. You actually feel programmed to say 'yes' and it happens before you even think properly about the request. For you, the most important thing to do is keep your mouth shut! Then when you open it, get in the habit of saying, 'I need some time to think about that, I'll get back to you' and give them a time frame.

The next step is to evaluate the request, but first we have to consider the other reasons why we say 'yes', which are feelings and skills.

2   Feelings. It's important to say yes to a request for positive reasons rather than to avoid negative ones. Say yes because you'll enjoy doing the job, it will serve a greater purpose, it will support the team, help the patients . . . whatever, as long as it's positive.

People often say 'yes' to avoid negative feelings in themselves or negative feelings in others. Their belief is that 'If I say no . . .

- I'll be letting people down
- they'll think I can't do my job properly
- although I know it's the right thing to say, I'll feel so guilty afterwards I may as well just say yes

- that'll mean I'll have some free time, and by staying busy I can avoid having to face the fact that I don't have much of a life outside of my workplace.'

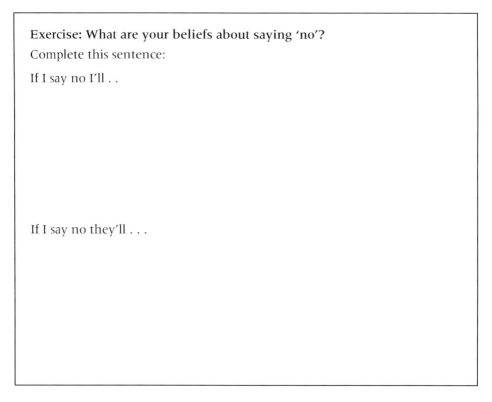

Exercise: What are your beliefs about saying 'no'?

Complete this sentence:

If I say no I'll . .

If I say no they'll . . .

The problem with these beliefs is that most of them involve guessing, usually incorrectly, other people's thoughts. What if you actually asked them, 'If I was to say no to doing a job, what would you think?' Usually people think that you are already working at full capacity but they may not know your reasons for saying no. In this case an explanation is in order, especially if you report to them. Just be honest; explain that you have too much on or that you don't have the appropriate resources or skills. Expect them to be understanding and you will be more likely to be assertive.

Sometimes people are manipulative using guilt. They behave coldly or sulk to either show you 'this is what it's like if I don't get my way' or because that is their default way of responding. The answer to this is to get used to being disliked occasionally. When you have made a decision with integrity that best serves the needs of the task, team or individual, remember the other person is responsible for their emotions, not you. Obviously explain to them the rationale behind your decision, help them with their feelings if that's appropriate and give them some time to cool off. If they continue with behaviour that is affecting their performance or that of the department, lead by compulsion and tell them such behaviour is not acceptable.

3 The right words. You actually want to say no but you just don't know the right words. Being blunt may be effective, but it can create bad feelings. The

important thing is for you to be comfortable with the words you use, so practise saying them aloud in a firm, confident voice to the mirror. For example:

'I have so many jobs to do at present that if I take on anything else, I won't be able to do my work to the appropriate standard.'

'I have so many jobs to do at present that if I take on anything else, I'll end up in the loony bin.'

'I appreciate what you are asking, however . . .' (give an explanation as to why you are turning down their request).

'Let me check exactly what it is you want me to do . . .' (feed back to them their request and the time frame for when it is due). 'Is that correct?' (wait for their answer). 'At the moment I have XYZ jobs to do. For me to do what you've requested, I'll need to put one/two of these jobs on hold. If you are OK with that, which one would you like me to put on hold?'

If someone persists with asking you to do something, just keep repeating what you have said. You don't have to come up with multiple explanations – for example, 'I don't have room to take on another project.' Alternatively declare the conversation over with 'I don't have anything more to add to this. Do you? OK then, I've got work to do.'

Evaluating requests

A request has been made and you've told them you need to think about it. Now you have to decide whether or not you want to do the job, so consider the following.

- Do you have the resources required, particularly time and energy, to do this job, *while* you meet all of your other commitments including looking after yourself?
- Do you want to do the job? Is it something you will enjoy? If the answer is yes, you may want to sacrifice another commitment in favour of this new opportunity.
- Even if you won't enjoy the job very much, will it serve you in the long term?
- Can anyone else do this job? If there are others available, and you don't want to do it, be strong and refuse. Don't become the person who gets the tag 'X will do it.' People will often take the path of least resistance which means going straight to you even if the task is not your responsibility.

Once you have made your decision, if it's a no, get comfortable with the right dialogue for you, connect with your bravery and say no. When you first start saying no, it takes a lot of courage so there are exercises in Chapter 7 called 'Building confidence' and 'Anchoring and assessing confidence' to help you develop that (pp. 54–5).

The other consequences most likely to arise when you start saying no are resistance from other people and your old habits asserting themselves.

In the face of resistance, give explanations and remain strong in your decision. Explain why you are changing how you take on jobs – for example, your work life is smothering your home life or you're losing the joy that you had in your work.

It's easy to fall back into old habits or patterns of behaviour. Accept setbacks and don't be hard on yourself. Put reminders in your environment to prompt your new behaviour like a note with 'no' written on it and a big smiley face. Recruit other people who support your change so they can check in with you and praise your progress. Finally, look for the positive results from saying no and accept them as a reward.

A note on 'time martyrs'

Some people say 'yes' to lots of activities or tasks so they can tell their friends and wait for their praise ('I don't know how you manage to do it all!') or sympathy ('You poor thing, you're so brave to battle on').

This attention from other people can become a game. It's like a tennis match. One person hits a complaint across the net; the other person returns a compliment or sympathy. Encouraging this type of game reinforces the negative behaviour of complaining. The person who often says 'It's OK, I'll manage' may be turning into a 'time martyr'.

This issue is raised because you may have someone on your team who falls into this category or you might even notice this condition has crept up on you. The key is to stop playing the game! Even off-hand complaints should be dealt with seriously. Don't let people off the hook with a flippant response. Ask them if they really are handling the workload or if they need any help or other resources. Be clear that it is their responsibility to inform you of any problems in getting the job done to the specified time frame and standard.

If people continue to make off-hand complaints that they don't really want you to act on, you have a couple of choices.

Request that they stop making these remarks because they make you concerned and confused about what's really going on as well as taking up a large amount of your time. Be prepared to reinforce this request.

If they keep complaining, take any extra work off them and give it to someone else.

Also, don't fall into the trap of regularly giving people additional work because they say 'yes'.

Your staff should be praised, thanked, complimented and rewarded for doing their standard jobs well, not just for doing something extra. Being paid doesn't equate to feeling appreciated and a vital part of any relationship is being appreciated.

Other tips for time investors

Say yes to something outside of work

Have you ever noticed how you can leave on time if there's something really important to get to? I knew a doctor who never ran late on a Wednesday night because he played competition tennis and he would have been letting his team down. Try marking in your diary a meeting in the evening and then tell others you have to get away on time for that. The meeting can be with your family or your bath-tub, but no-one else has to know that. Just treat it as a very important thing you need to do.

Stop paper shuffling

Every time you pick up a piece of paper, put a red tick on it. After you have handled it a dozen times and can hardly read it for red ticks, you will take action.

To-do lists and the 3-Ds strategy

Often there are things to do on our lists that just get copied over to the next day's list. When you next see one of these offending activities, do it, delegate it or dump it.

1 Do it. If it's a huge task, break it down into smaller chunks that are more appealing to do. To get you started, use a cooking timer and set it for 10 minutes. Either you will invest a minimum of 10 minutes on it or you will set the timer for another 10 minutes as it's not as bad as you expected.
2 Delegate it. If someone else can do the job, either from within the business or externally, give the job to them. Buying in skills is often cheaper when compared to the amount of time wasted by you thinking about the job that never gets done. Delegation is covered in detail in Chapter 9 (p. 71).
3 Dump it. Take it off the list and don't bother doing it. Often this is the case with reading for professional development. If you have piles of papers or journals for reading that you still haven't got to, pack them in a box, tape it up, write the date six months away on the top and if you haven't opened it by then, recycle the lot. Most of what you are throwing away can be accessed on the internet anyway.

Close your office door

This avoids you being distracted by what's happening outside and tells others that you are not to be disturbed. One doctor I knew had a circular sign like a clock pie-chart with an arrow that she could point to different sections such as 'patients', 'do not disturb' and 'come in'. If people ask 'Can I interrupt you?', that's often broken your train of thought anyway. So let them know when they can see you, without having to ask you.

Suggested learning outcomes and action points

1 Understand the 'YOW' question and how to use it for problem analysis and to create solutions.
2 Know how to apply Stephen Covey's Time Management Matrix for prioritising and categorising activities.
3 Know how to apply the Time-Usage Continuum for prioritising activities; be aware of the language you use when referring to activities (is an activity a 'waste' or an 'investment' of time?) and use it as a trigger for action.
4 If you haven't already done so, do the exercises on 'What you do with your time', 'In an ideal world!' and 'Inspiration'.

5 Explore what underlies your difficulty with saying 'no' to others and with prioritising yourself.

Reference

1 Covey S. *The Seven Habits of Highly Effective People*. 1st ed. New York: Simon & Schuster; 1990.

Further reading

• Harvard Business School Press. *Time Management – Increase Your Personal Productivity and Effectiveness*. Boston: Harvard Business School Publishing Corporation; 2005.
• Newman S. *The Book of No: 250 Ways to Say It – and Mean It and Stop People-pleasing Forever*. London: McGraw-Hill Publishing Co; 2006.

Chapter 3

Leadership model

'What does a leader actually do?'

There are obvious 'leaders' in primary care such as the business owners, practice managers and team leaders. However, we believe anyone who has a strategic, supportive or teaching role needs leadership skills irrespective of their official position.

The action-centred leadership model

A useful starting point for developing leadership skills is to consider a model that can be applied to all situations. One of the most enduring and simple models is the action-centred leadership (ACL) model created by John Adair in the 1960s. He developed and tested this model while working at the Royal Military Academy Sandhurst and the model was eventually adopted as the core of their leadership training. It was later rolled out to the other armed forces and has since been taught in numerous environments including corporate, social development and higher education. *See* Figure 3.1.

This model illustrates the relationship between the needs of the task, team and individual. Crucially, it notes that they are interconnected and an effective leader therefore monitors all three elements and adjusts their focus accordingly. A leader's prime goal is the achievement of the task, hence its position at the top of the diagram. The team and individual needs should then be met as best as possible to support the task.

The task

The term 'task' refers to those things that must be achieved whether it is in the short, medium or long term.

A long-term task could include: acquiring new premises to expand a general practice or changing the management team structure.

Medium-term tasks could include: implementing a new pay system, ensuring the professional development of new nurses or adding a new partner to a practice.

Short-term tasks could include: ensuring all patients are treated to a standard of excellence on a daily basis, hygiene standards are maintained minute by minute or trainees have one formal training event per week.

The team

Your role will determine whether you are the leader of a multidisciplinary or single discipline team. For example, a practice manager has the responsibility of patient care by maximising how well all of the teams perform together. The nursing team

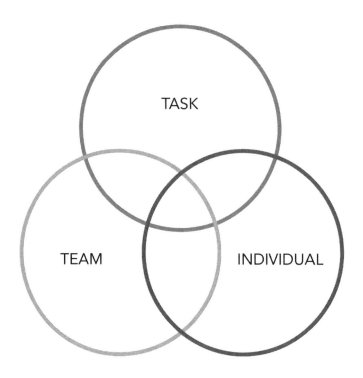

Figure 3.1 ACL model – three overlapping circles of needs.[1]

leader however will only lead their team and be a liaison with other management staff.

The leader of a team must ensure that the appropriate resources are available and are utilised as well as develop the performance of the team as a unit and not simply as a group of individuals. Teambuilding skills are therefore a key element of leadership capability.

The individual

Human needs have been studied for decades with probably the best-known research conducted by Abraham Maslow in 1943. The result was Maslow's Hierarchy of Needs[2] which indicates that people must meet their most 'basic needs' such as food, shelter and security before pursuing 'higher needs' such as sense of belonging, self-esteem, recognition and self-actualisation. There are many other needs which drive behaviour such as cooperation, honesty, balance, respect, freedom, care, and inclusion, to name a few.

As the leader, it is your job to be aware that these needs may surface at any time. Taking the view that all behaviour is an expression of a person trying to get their needs met brings a whole new light to understanding people's behaviour. This does not mean, however, that all behaviour is necessarily appropriate.

As individuals try to meet their needs, their behaviour may change or be perceived as difficult. Someone seeking accuracy and order may struggle with effective delegation. Similarly, someone needing recognition may appear to be irritable if they do not receive praise.

While people are working to have their needs met they are invariably less able to be creative and focused on the task and hence their performance will be lessened. As the leader's focus is achievement of the task they must address any behaviour that is detrimental to the individual or team's performance. Specifically identifying the needs driving unhelpful behaviours will allow you to get to the root of the problem.

In addition to needs, learning style preferences, levels of knowledge, skills and strengths will also vary between individuals. Knowing these gives the leader greater potential to bring out the best performance in each individual.

Exercise: Applying the ACL model

Consider a leadership situation that you are currently involved in. What are or might be the needs of the task?

Which teams are involved, e.g. the nursing team, the admin team? What are or might be the needs of each individual team?

What are or might be the needs of the greater practice team?

What are or might be the needs of the individuals?

The basic leadership functions

John Adair notes that leaders should be capable of six basic leadership functions and their associated activities, which I have elaborated on below. There are though a few things to keep in mind beforehand.

Leaders at different levels in a business find they have to satisfy these functions in different proportions. You may not even have to do some of these functions but be aware of what is happening in those areas as it affects you and your team. If you are the business owner or manager you will be doing a lot of planning and initiating, whereas a team leader who needs leadership capability will be doing a larger proportion of controlling and supporting.

These leadership functions also don't have to be done by you alone. A lot of them are best done in collaboration with your colleagues, staff and customers as you tap a rich source of information and also show that their opinions are valuable to you.

Ideally the decisions you make as a leader will follow information gathering from other people and sources. For those in a large business you have multiple colleagues to call upon. Even if you are a single-handed general practitioner and you are the leader and the management, you can seek input from the staff that you trust, your patients, family, friends and members of your professional network. You could also speak with a coach or mentor who could provide an independent perspective.

As you read through the following functions and actions, consider:

- what you are really good at and do more of it
- what you are OK at and either get better at it or delegate it
- what you are not good at and either improve to the minimal level that your role requires or delegate it.

1 Planning

a Seek all available information from relevant people including your staff, customers (patients, the health authority), trust representatives and those who are politically aware.
b Define vision, group/team task, purpose or goals, remembering this may be the ultimate purpose of the general practice (e.g. creating and maintaining excellent health in the community; getting patient satisfaction surveys completed by a deadline).
c Make a workable plan in conjunction with the relevant people to achieve the goal.

2 Initiating

a Brief the group/team on the goals and the strategy.
b Explain why the goals or strategy are necessary, specifying the benefits to be gained or negative consequences to be avoided.
c Allocate tasks to group members ensuring as far as possible that each individual utilises their strengths.
d Set group standards for behaviour, performance and note the steps toward the end goal.

3 Controlling

a Maintain group standards.
b Influence tempo (i.e. speed up the pace if it is too slow or reflecting complacency and slow the pace if people are acting too quickly without due consideration).
c Ensure all actions are taken towards meeting objectives (i.e. preventing postponement or avoidance of actions). If avoidance is occurring, the needs of the individuals and team/group should be explored to identify the obstacles to progress.
d Keep discussion relevant to keep people interested and prevent time wasting.

e   Steer the group to action/decision. If a consensus cannot be reached having reviewed all available information, it will be up to the leader to make a decision.

4 Supporting

a   Accept people and appreciate their contribution.
b   Encourage the team and individuals.
c   Discipline the team and individuals as needed to maintain standards and progress.
d   Create a sense of purpose and accountability in the group/team.
e   Reconcile disagreements or encourage others to explore them and to reach a resolution.

5 Informing

a   Clarify the task and plan once it has been initiated.
b   Provide new information to the group so they are aware of the big picture. People rarely complain about knowing detail, but they will complain about not being informed.
c   Receive information from the group so you are able to review progress in relation to the goal as well as the effectiveness of strategy.
d   Summarise suggestions and ideas coherently so that you can present information in an easy-to-understand manner. As a manager, you will need to do this for your direct reports and your supervisor.

6 Evaluating

a   Check the feasibility of ideas and ensure all of the concerns and information are aired and debated.
b   Test the consequences of a proposed solution by imagining the solution has already been implemented and exploring the result.
c   Evaluate group/team performance and make appropriate changes if the team is not performing to the desired standard.
d   Help the group to evaluate its own performance against standards.

To help you remember these functions, just think you have to be a 'PICSIE' to lead.

Exercise: Applying the PICSIE

Consider a leadership situation that you are currently involved in.

- What planning steps have been done and what still needs to be done?
- What initiating steps have been done and what still needs to be done?
- What controlling steps have been done and what still needs to be done?
- What supporting steps have been done and what still needs to be done?
- What informing steps have been done and what still needs to be done?
- What evaluating steps have been done and what still needs to be done?

Suggested learning outcomes and action points

1 Understand the Adair action-centred leadership model.
2 Be able to review a leadership situation and consider what the needs are for the task, team and individuals.
3 Understand what is involved in the six key functions of a leader: planning, initiating, controlling, supporting, informing and evaluating (PICSIE).
4 If you haven't already done so, do the exercises 'Applying the ACL model' and 'Applying the PICSIE'.

References

1 Adair J. *Effective Leadership Development*. London: The Chartered Institute of Personnel and Development; 2006.
2 Maslow A. *Motivation and Personality*. New York: Harper; 1954.

Further reading

• Blanchard K, Zigarmi P, Zigarmi D. *Leadership and the One Minute Manager*. London: HarperCollins, 2004.

Chapter 4

Leadership styles and techniques

'What are the different ways to lead and how do I know when to use a particular style?'

Defining leadership

At this stage, you know what to focus on and the activities you need to be capable of achieving to be an effective leader. But what happens on a practical level? If you've planned a strategy, do you just tell people what to do and expect them to do it? Do you seek their input or do you persuade them before going into action?

What varies here is the style of leadership. It's about 'how' you get people to follow your lead. This depends on:

- the nature and demands of the task
- the time frame available to achieve the task
- the practical skill level of the team and individuals involved
- the commitment and motivation level of the team and individuals involved
- your leadership goals, i.e. if your goal is to empower your team and create a greater sense of responsibility and motivation, then leading by enabling instead of leading by compulsion will allow you to more easily meet that goal, but more on this later.

People often ask 'what is the best style?'

The *best* style is **the one that gets the job done while balancing task achievement with the relationships involved.** Usually a combination of styles is most effective in achieving a result; however, the choice of style(s) depends on the situation.

An excellent definition of leadership can be found in the Defence Leadership Handbook © DLC which states:

> Leadership is visionary; it is the projection of personality and character to inspire people to achieve the desired outcome. There is no prescription of leadership and no prescribed style of leader. Leadership is a combination of example, persuasion and compulsion dependent on the situation. It should aim to transform and be underpinned by individual skills and an enabling philosophy. The successful leader is an individual who understands himself/herself, the organisation, the environment in which they operate and the people that they are privileged to lead.[1]

This definition reveals the features of an effective leader and the styles that can be used.

Features of leaders

The three fundamental features are:

1 An *external awareness* (i.e. they understand the organisation, the environment in which they operate, the people they lead and the situation in which they are required to lead).
2 An *internal awareness* (i.e. they understand themselves, know their individual skills, have an enabling philosophy and a sense of privilege to be in their position).
3 The *willingness to take action* (i.e. they actively project their personality and character to inspire people to achieve the desired outcome and can lead using different styles).

Styles

The five leadership styles (*see* Figure 4.1) are:

1 Leading by example. This means that you demonstrate to your staff, colleagues and/or boss the standards of performance and behaviour you want them to reflect.
2 Leading by persuasion. This means appealing to people's logic, values, emotions and needs in order for them to behave or perform in a manner that will support achievement of the task.

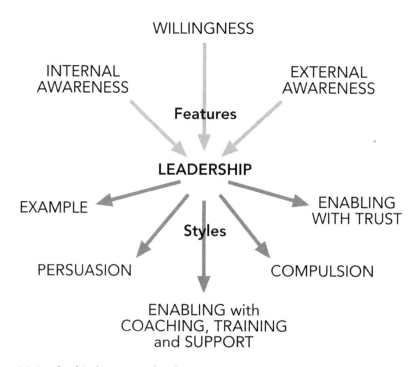

Figure 4.1 Leadership features and styles.

3   Leading by compulsion. This involves giving direct instructions without seeking the person's input or telling someone it is compulsory for them to perform to a certain standard or to behave in a given way.

Leading by an enabling philosophy which in practical terms involves:

4   Leading by enabling with coaching, training and support. This involves helping others learn through coaching, training and ensuring that they know you will support them by providing resources or removing obstacles to their development. These obstacles can be situational such as preventing another staff member from inhibiting newcomers' development or they can be innate such as a lack of confidence.
5   Leading by enabling with trust. This involves giving people the freedom to do a task where the responsibility and accountability for the end result is largely if not all theirs.

Consider which leadership styles could be used in the following scenario.

Inducting a new receptionist

The practice manager or the reception team leader are the ones most likely to be involved in this process and their priorities will be to:

- evaluate the level of her knowledge on topics from computer skills to patient confidentiality
- understand how she prefers to learn (i.e. reading, being told, shown or practising)
- evaluate how enthusiastic and engaged she is.

The leader will be able to use many styles depending on the situation. She will lead by:

- example to demonstrate the practice standards of efficacy and behaviour
- persuasion to explain why certain operating procedures exist
- enabling through coaching, training and trust for learning tasks and building confidence.

Leading by compulsion may be required if the receptionist refuses to work according to the practice protocols or breaches behaviour standards. Hopefully this will not occur.

Understanding the features of leaders

There has been a great deal of discussion with very little agreement over many years about the 'qualities' of leaders. Essentially, developing leadership capability is *not* about focusing on developing certain qualities. Instead, strong leaders develop attitudes, skills and areas of awareness in line with their strengths.

Remember, 'there is no prescription of leadership and no prescribed style of leader'. Don't try to be someone that you are not. You will be awkward, uncomfortable and unfocused as you think more about how you appear than what you are doing. Just think for a moment about some famous leaders; they are often religious, military, business or political leaders. Commonly identified leaders are Sir Winston Churchill, Mahatma Gandhi, Sir Richard Branson, General Napoleon Bonaparte and Reverend Martin Luther King Jr. Think for a moment about their personalities and notice the differences. There are some similarities in what they do but their personalities are certainly dissimilar.

Nevertheless, personal integrity is the one vital common denominator quality of any great leader.

A person that accepts a leadership position to boost their ego, wield a sense of superiority and impose their prejudices on others is not going to be a truly great leader. They may experience success in some form but typically their staff will not be listened to, or be given responsibility, recognition or the freedom to be inventive and grow. It is most likely that staff will eventually rebel and leave.

Strong personal integrity will result in a leader that is driven by values and a desire to create a truly great healthcare service that will evolve long after they have gone. In short, their willingness to be a leader will be great and consequently they will be adaptable and flexible in the methods they use to achieve that. They will demand accountability, honesty, open-mindedness and involvement from their staff, their colleagues and their patients. Yes, patients too must be held accountable for their involvement in their care and how they interact with the providers of the service. Leaders will not tolerate compromises in standards of service or behaviour and they will always be seeking improvements, though they will not implement change unless it is necessary.

A leader must be emotionally strong to do these things. Reminding yourself of the reasons that you took the position can help you tap into your integrity and inspire you.

Exercise: Why do you want a leadership role?

Take a few minutes now to write down the reasons you want to be a leader. What do you want to change? What do you want to create? What legacy do you want to leave? What do you want people to say about you as a leader? What else made you take on this role?

External awareness

The organisation

You must understand the history, current state and future goals of the organisation that you lead. This allows you to appreciate the existing culture and feelings of the people you are leading as well as knowing the direction in which the organisation is moving.

Also be sure that you know how your organisation fits in the bigger picture of the health sector and your community. A general practice will probably have direct contact with other practices that it commissions services from, a health trust at 'local' level and the Department of Health. It is also important to be aware of district and city councils and local police, in the event of building modifications or other developments around you that may have an impact on access for patients or service delivery.

The environment

The 'environment' includes the *physical, political, economic* and *social* environments in which the practice exists. All environments must be considered in their current context as well as the changes that the future may bring. Even if the changes are not expected to occur for 10 years (e.g. increasing demand on rehabilitation services due to an ageing population), the plans to accommodate such change may need to be prepared and initiated now.

The *physical* environment requires consideration of several components.

- How much space do people have to work in? Are people cramped and if so do they work effectively in that environment?
- Does it take staff a long time to move between departments or key people? This will impact how swiftly and easily information can flow.
- What is the size of the geographic area across which your team and customers are placed? Does this mean more time is needed for travel to attend meetings? Would telephone conferencing or more efficient information technology reduce time wasted and frustration for staff?
- What kind of equipment is available and used by staff? If the workspace that your staff occupies is tired and unkept, it may have a negative impact on their mood and productivity. Think also of how frustrating it is to work with computers that regularly crash or are extremely slow.

A special note: Don't expect that making changes in work conditions will necessarily make people feel more satisfied at work. Good conditions will prevent them from feeling dissatisfied, which is equally important because then you have a foundation upon which to build job satisfaction and realise an improvement in engagement at work. Remember the Herzberg experiments of Chapter 1.

The most valuable thing to do in reviewing the physical environment is to ask the staff for their input. They will soon identify what's helping and hindering them.

The *political* environment has an impact on patients' expectations, staff morale and an organisation's plans.

If governments regularly tell patients that their doctors should be available 24 hours a day, seven days a week, then that is the expectation for the general practice. If staff regularly hear that there will be funding cuts for their hospital they may begin to fear for their jobs and morale could suffer.

A practice or hospital that is planning their future over the next 10 years must also bear in mind what the potential changes are for the healthcare sector. Will there be more privatisation? Will there be stricter controls by government on how general practices earn money? What scenarios are likely?

The *economic* environment will impact the amount and quality of resources available for patients and staff. Simplifying and standardising processes can lead to savings and begins with talking to frontline staff to find out where time is wasted or where inefficiencies arise. There are only two ways to make processes more efficient: either eliminate a step in the process or ensure each step is performed as close to 100% accurately more often. Using processes already proven in other organisations and tweaking them to fit yours is a great time saver and a way to rapidly boost efficiency. Consider the programmes from the Institute for Healthcare Improvement[2] such as the 100,000 Lives Campaign and the lean production principles of the Toyota Production System in the manufacture of cars.

When planning for the future, consider what the economic needs will be for your organisation. As a minimum you will need to view:

- the current state of the facilities and the improvements that are needed
- new services to add or existing ones to be enhanced
- further training that staff may need with changing or developing roles.

Try being idealistic and make a wish list. Then compare your list with the projected budget and decide what you can afford. You may not be able to do all of the things on your wish list, but they may be sufficiently inspiring to allow you to adopt new strategies and ways of working in order to increase your income to pursue your list. Conversely you may choose to take a lower income in favour of investing in additional staff, thus freeing you to pursue other interests.

The *social* environment will influence the health of a community and hence the type and level of demand for clinical and social care. Each community will also have expectations on the services that should be provided and when and how they can be accessed. Once these facts are known, the organisation can plan to manage unrealistic expectations and accurately tailor their clinical services to their patients.

The people

Understanding the people you are leading involves getting to know them – for example, knowing their strengths, values, ambitions, 'usual' behaviour in relation to their personality type, how they behave under pressure and their learning style. This may seem like a lot of information but the more that you know, the stronger your relationships and position of influence will be.

You can elicit this information formally or informally. Getting to know a person well goes beyond superficial chatting, which some people may find intimidating. If this is the case, doing this work in a group during a meeting specifically for development will usually make people more comfortable. Set the scene by explaining what you hope to achieve by understanding each other better in terms of communication, finding common ground and helping people to work in areas that are their strengths. An external facilitator may be useful to initiate this process so that the management team or business owner is viewed as part of the team.

The following formal assessments can be used.

- The StrengthsFinder Profile by Buckingham and Clifton.[3] This is an online assessment for individuals that considers 34 themes of strengths such as empathy, developer, analytical and learner. To complete the assessment you need a 'code' number which comes with the book *Now, Discover Your Strengths.*
- Myers-Briggs Type Indicator for individual personality typing. The person administering this assessment will have a formal qualification. See the website www.myersbriggs.org for a list of organisations that provide training.[4]
- Belbin® is a well-accepted approach to identify team roles and assessments that can be purchased at www.belbin.com/onlinetest.htm.[5] For general information *see* Chapter 11 (p. 106).
- For learning styles there appears to be no formal regulation when undertaking such assessments. There are several available online, some of which are free. Learning about neuro-linguistic programming (NLP) will also give you a good understanding of learning styles.

The results of any of these assessments do not intend to set in stone how a person behaves; rather they provide a platform for discussion. The differences that we all have can often make communication and understanding really difficult. Airing these differences allows people to view situations from others' perspectives and to look at ways they can behave differently to make working together less stressful and communication more effective.

Most people have a need for recognition and contribution. Having their opinion valued just by being asked and acknowledged is a great way of engaging people, as is learning what is working and what isn't at the frontline of your organisation. A formal process to capture people's input is invaluable, even if it is just a routine part of regular staff meetings. Try therefore to avoid putting if off to deal with other, apparently more pressing issues. As a leader you will probably have an opinion on most issues but in keeping with your integrity you must always be prepared to listen to other perspectives, data and suggestions.

More on learning styles

Knowing the various ways by which we learn will allow you to be more effective when leading by coaching, training or persuading. Generally people have a preferred style, so when presenting to a group, use as many styles as possible. If you are working with one individual, then identifying their specific preferences will help you with your approach.

Visual learners learn through seeing, so enjoy diagrams, charts, videos and the expressions of the teacher. They will often take notes so they have a visual reference for later. If ever you feel like saying 'you don't need to write this down', as they reach for a pen, then think again.

Auditory learners learn through listening so enjoy lectures, discussions and talking things through. They may find notes distracting or unnecessary so may ignore your carefully prepared handout.

Tactile or kinaesthetic learners learn by doing, touching or moving so are very hands-on. They are the 'let me have a go' types and only then do they feel confident they have learned.

Active learners like to do something with the information they have received so they may discuss it, apply it or explain it to others. They naturally like learning in groups.

Reflective learners tend to think quietly about the information before doing any anything, so like to learn alone.

Sequential learners like to learn one step at a time and may become confused if your presentation or conversation jumps around.

Global learners like to know the big picture first and may not understand the various steps as you present. Once accomplished, it all comes together in a flash for them.

When you are presenting to a *group* with a mix of these styles, do the following to be effective:

- Present information using diagrams where possible and bullet points.
- Speak with energy; don't bore your auditory learners by talking in a monotone.
- If you are teaching a skill allow time for people to practise.
- Don't push everyone to be engaged in the learning immediately; your reflective listeners may become stressed.
- Give the big picture of the topic first and then fill in the detail.

When you are working with an *individual*, talk about the topic with them, let them take notes, ask if diagrams or illustrations would be helpful and allow them to practise if they want to. If they become quiet after you explain something, check if they are reflecting, are confused or need more information. Give them the big picture or purpose behind what you are going to be working on first and then be sequential in your teaching.

The situation

The nature and demands of the task and the time frame available to achieve the task will determine which leadership styles you use. For example, a cardiac arrest situation will require you to take control and act within a very short time frame. Leading by compulsion will therefore be appropriate. Alternatively, teaching communication skills over several weeks while developing that person's confidence and creativity will be better served by leading with coaching, training and support.

How to develop external awareness

The starting point is knowing what you need to learn and then finding the people or resources to give you that knowledge.

When you take a leadership role in a new environment allow yourself the time to learn this information. Maintaining this level of knowledge and awareness can then be done informally through conversation or formally through conferences, meetings and reviews (interviews or questionnaires) with staff, local and regional policy makers and customers (patients, other practices and organisations).

Exercise: Increasing your external awareness

List three resources (such as people and websites) that could increase your awareness and understanding of:

- the organisation

- the physical environment

- the political environment

- the economic environment

- the social environment

- the people.

Note, alongside the names, when and how you will make first contact with them, how you will maintain contact and how frequently you will do this. It is best to systemise the regular contact you want to keep, otherwise it may be forgotten. Have a regular slot marked out in your diary to maintain your relationships, whether it is over coffee, at formal meetings or with a phone call.

Internal awareness

Internal awareness means knowing:

- your values and needs (note: there is an exercise for this in Chapter 5, 'Identifying your needs and values, p. 42).
- what drives your behaviour
- your strengths (so that you can develop them further) and your weaknesses (so that you can manage them)
- your personality so that you understand how you interact with the world and behave under pressure and how that affects other people
- your emotions and attitude in a given situation
- your overall level of health and how you are coping.

Let's consider these in turn.

What drives your behaviour?

This is strongly affected by your values and needs as well as whether you move 'away' from a painful situation or move 'toward' a more pleasurable situation.

Exercise: Do you move away from pain or move toward pleasure?

Think back to the times in your life when you have made a change such as quitting jobs, moving house, changing a subject you were studying . . . any kind of change.

When you think about those times, were you in an acceptable situation and then decided to move toward a more positive experience or did you only make a change when your situation became so bad that you couldn't stand it?

This knowledge can be applied when you need motivation to make a change. Create a picture of the painful results of not changing and the positive results of making the change. Make the richest picture of the pain or pleasure that drives you the most. Consider the results in terms of how you, your customers, your team and the organisation will be affected physically, mentally, financially, in relationships, in service provision and career development.

Your strengths and weaknesses

Knowing your strengths, which is also discussed in more detail in Chapter 10, is one of the most valuable pieces of knowledge to have. One of the best definitions for strengths comes from authors Buckingham and Clifton in the book *Now, Discover Your Strengths*.[3] They define strengths as: 'consistent, near perfect performance in an activity that brings positive outcome'. These activities generally come quite naturally to you.

Also think of how enthusiastic you feel when you know that you are going to do something that you are good at, compared with doing something that you are not very good at. There's usually a lot less enthusiasm, coupled with resistance, when you are not doing things you are strong at. The studies by Buckingham and Clifton on strengths and weaknesses have led them to recommend that people focus on developing their strengths and manage their areas of weakness. For most people, this is a welcome relief.

One of my clients described that her strongest leadership styles were leading by persuasion and example and she really disliked leading by compulsion. She knew she was very good at empathising, presenting a good argument and inspiring people. To be a more effective leader she chose to invest more time and energy in doing those things she already did well and as a result she had fewer events which required her to lead by compulsion. She also noted the relief and boosted energy levels among her staff when she told them in a meeting that they would be just focusing on what they did well and how to develop those areas. Everyone perked up, felt positive and they had a more productive meeting.

Your personality

Personality-type assessments are not designed to put you in a category that suggests you can't change your ways. They are designed to identify trends in how you think and behave and what motivates you. They should open up discussion about the results of an assessment to explore how different elements impact on different situations.

Probably the most famous assessment is the Myers-Briggs Type Indicator®. There are others however such as the 'PIAV' (personal interests, attitudes and values), 'DISC' (dominance, influence, steadiness and conscientiousness) and '16PF' (personality factors). Yet others are more specific to team behaviour such as 'FIRO-B'® (Fundamental Interpersonal Relations Orientation-Behavior™). Any internet search engine will reveal multiple organisations and individuals that provide these assessments.

Your emotions and attitude in a given situation

Self-awareness of your attitude, which results from your thoughts and feelings, allows you to regulate your behaviour and help address any issues that may come up for you. A useful tip to remember is that every emotion is preceded by a thought. This may come as a surprise, but once you test this idea you will become more alert to how your thoughts affect your feelings.

For example, I used to feel frustrated with some of my physiotherapy patients when I took their history and they digressed into irrelevant details. I realised I was thinking: 'Just get on with the story; can't you stick with the facts?' Once I was thinking like this, my mood would change and I didn't enjoy the work. So I changed my thoughts. As soon as I felt the frustration rising in me, I would think: 'This must be really hard for them.' As a result I felt compassionate instead. If your thoughts give you negative emotions then identify which thoughts would put you in a more positive state to better handle the situation.

Your attitude, which reflects your beliefs, similarly has an enormous impact on your behaviour. If you believe that you are privileged to lead others, you will convey a sense of gratitude and respect to them and act accordingly. Compare this to the actions that would stem from a leader that is reluctant to be in their position or wants to be a leader to make themselves feel superior. Have you ever worked for a poor leader? Chances are that other people's opinions and suggestions were either ignored or taken on without being properly evaluated. The leader may have been a dictator or a pushover, all of which have a negative impact on the team and its task.

Your overall level of health and how you are coping

If you wish to remain in a leadership position for a long time, you must learn to invest in your physical and mental health. This requires time. If you already set aside time for exercise, prayer, meditation or hobbies that give you the opportunity to switch off from work and invest in yourself, then you need to protect that time. You may find that as your work intensifies, you need to be even stronger with yourself in saying no to people who try to invade those times.

If you don't regularly do any activities to recharge your batteries then try to recognise if you are feeling more irritable, tired, intolerant, or if you are getting ill more often. Also pay attention to feedback from friends and family as others can often see subtle changes in you, before you do.

Willingness to take action

As a leader you must be willing to do what is necessary to achieve the task at hand while balancing the needs of the individuals and teams involved. Your level of willingness will be influenced by a number of things, namely:

- your personal integrity and desire to provide excellent healthcare
- the strength of your vision for the future and your ability to see the light at the end of the tunnel when times are tough
- your skill level and confidence for developing awareness and using different leadership styles
- your self-esteem, which will enable you to project your personality so you don't feel you must 'be someone else' to be a great leader
- your understanding of your own strengths and the ability to find and develop opportunities to use them.

Having these will mean that, in practical terms, you:

- have the confidence to state, support and, if necessary, defend your strategies and judgements because you know what is best for the immediate situation and the long-term vision
- have the ability to inspire others with your vision
- are on the lookout for development opportunities for yourself and others
- have the confidence to seek input from others, even in unrelated industries, without feeling like you should know it all
- have the desire to be held accountable for goals and standards, in order to get results and to create the right culture in your organisation
- utilise your strengths on a daily basis.

If at any time in your career you feel that your confidence, self-esteem, skill level or knowledge is not at a level that makes you a great leader, then seek support. This can be done on a one-to-one basis or in groups via coaching, training, mentoring and learning sets. The latter is a group of peers that meet regularly to offer counsel and support.

If you find that issues arise from your past because of the demands or nature of your work, consider counselling also; there is no stigma in wanting to better yourself. You are taking positive steps to develop for your own good and for the good of others. Imagine the cost of not taking this action. Your talents and gifts may be lost from the medical world and at a cost to your personal well-being.

What is your leadership preference?

The quiz in Table 4.1 will get you thinking about your current and favoured leadership styles.

Table 4.1 What is your leadership preference?

	Yes/agree	No/disagree
Example		
What I do is more important than what I say.		
I expect others to do as I do.		
People look to me to see how I respond to events and ideas.		
TOTAL	Yes/agree	/3
Persuasion		
I find it easy to understand how other people are feeling.		
I like presenting an argument to win people over.		
People come to me to understand the different sides to and facts around a decision or proposal.		
TOTAL	Yes/agree	/3
Compulsion		
I tend to tell people what to do without waiting for their input.		
I tend to take charge in a crisis and expect people to do as I say.		
I am completely comfortable telling people what they can and can't do.		
TOTAL	Yes/agree	/3
Enabling with coaching, training and support		
I like helping people develop professionally and personally.		
People come to me for emotional support and to use me as a resource.		
People tell me I am a good teacher or that they've learned a lot from me.		
TOTAL	Yes/agree	/3
Enabling with trust		
I like it when 'my students' become independent and confident in their work.		
The people I train and coach know they'll be autonomous as soon as possible.		
I enjoy delegating and giving people the opportunity to demonstrate their skills.		
TOTAL	Yes/agree	/3

Exercise: How effective is your style?

Now that you know your preferred style, consider how effective it is for you in your workplace.

- What challenging leadership situations have you been in during the past six months?

- Which ones were you not as effective or successful in as you would have liked?
- Which of your non-preferred styles might have been more effective?
- Which of your preferred styles could you have used more of to be more effective?

It's important for you to lead according to your preferred style, as you will probably be most effective with that, but you must also be competent in the other styles.

If you don't/can't lead by example, and you set a negative example, you risk having your staff doing the same.

If you don't/can't lead by persuasion you will have difficulty implementing changes that require a good explanation because you will be less likely to have the support of your staff.

If you don't/can't lead by compulsion you may struggle when you have to handle difficult behaviour by staff. Compulsion becomes less of a necessity as you become better at leading using the other techniques.

If you don't/can't lead by enabling with coaching, training and support you will need to either delegate this role to a colleague or use external services. Without this, staff skill levels will stagnate and they may become disillusioned with the lack of development opportunities.

If you don't/can't lead by enabling with trust you will have great difficulty delegating and end up feeling overwhelmed by the workload as you try to do everything yourself.

When you need to use styles that are not your preference consider the skills that you need as well as your emotions and thoughts associated with those styles. If the thought of leading by compulsion fills you with terror, or leading by coaching makes you feel irritated, then you must address those emotions so that you are in a positive state as you apply the skills. How to do this is covered in detail in the coming chapters.

Accountability

With so many leaders and so much enabling, empowering and input being sought from other staff, who has the final say? Who is accountable?

In a general practice it is those who own the business that have the final say. They have invested their money; they are the ones who will be severely impacted financially if the business fails; they will probably be involved in any legal action against the practice; and so ultimately they are the decision makers on how their business runs. This includes not only the business operations but the clinical and behavioural standards to which they and their staff must adhere.

This does not mean the practice is run purely by compulsion where staff are simply told what to do and expected to do it. Wise leaders will seek input from those with the relevant knowledge, which means all of the staff and the customers. They also know that having a workforce of active and enthusiastic participants creates an enjoyable workplace, a positive atmosphere and improves their bottom line.

Ground rules

When you are enabling your staff and encouraging them to contribute it is essential that they know exactly what their responsibilities are and how they link with the responsibilities of the management team. Ideally these ground rules are defined in their job description and therefore are part of their employment contract. If they are not already part of their contract you cannot change them without consulting them. To ensure that you comply with employment law while making changes, use a human resources consultancy or employment law solicitor. You may need to implement a formal consultation period in which you negotiate the new standards.

Once formed, these ground rules are an agreed reference point for the leaders and staff. They are particularly useful when a staff member fails to meet their responsibilities or inappropriately attempts to take over another person's responsibilities. Likewise, if the management team fails to meet their responsibilities the staff may remind them of the ground rules.

For example, some of a practice partner's responsibilities might include:

- eight clinical sessions per week
- supporting the practice manager in their human resources role
- active involvement in decision making on business strategy and development, personnel development and patient care
- enforcing practice standards and implementation of new decisions.

Some of a receptionist's responsibilities might include:

- greeting patients politely and positively at the front desk
- scheduling appointments by phone and face to face
- active involvement in making suggestions to improve business operations, patient care and personnel development
- contributing to developing staff relations by behaving in a supportive and respectful manner to all other staff.

Whatever the job or responsibility, people are happier when they know what to do, by when and to what standard. Having ground rules can cement the way people work and facilitate trust.

Suggested learning outcomes and action points

1 Know how to increase your external awareness to improve your leadership capability.
2 Select one area of your external awareness to develop that would make you a better leader if you knew more about it and create an action plan to increase your knowledge.
3 Know how to increase your internal awareness to improve your leadership capability.
4 Take a StrengthsFinder or personality-type assessment.
5 Know the five leadership styles and explore your own real-life situations to identify the most appropriate styles to use.

6 Know your leadership style preferences and create an action plan to further develop your strengths and an action plan to improve at the styles you are not strong at.

References

1 Royal Air Force. Extract from *Defence Leadership Handbook* © DLC: http://raf.mod.uk/leadershipcentre/definition.html
2 Institute for Healthcare Improvement: www.ihi.org
3 Buckingham M, Clifton D. *Now, Discover your Strengths*. London: Pocket Books; 2005.
4 www.myersbriggs.org
5 www.belbin.com/onlinetest.htm

Further reading

- *Going Lean in Health Care* (White Paper): www.ihi.org/IHI/Results/WhitePapers/

Chapter 5

Leading by example

When what you do is more important than what you say.

When to use this style

Imagine you are a locum doctor sharing a treatment room and are told to maintain the room in a particular state of cleanliness by the doctor with whom you share, who is also one of the partners. The partner however always leaves the room in a state below the standard that is commonly demanded. You will probably notice that you begin to feel resentment toward the partner who doesn't follow the rules.

Or imagine you have just joined the reception team and the team leader has told you how important it is to be punctual to meetings. She then repeatedly arrives 10 minutes late. What would you think? You probably wouldn't believe it is important to be on time to those meetings and you might even question other things that she says, maybe even her integrity.

In both situations it is the example that carries the message to others, not the words. Leading by example reflects the adage 'actions speak louder than words' and is one of the most powerful styles of leadership.

In any leadership situation, ask yourself, 'What do my actions tell those around me?'
Consider these further examples.

1　Everyone in your general practice is weary from implementing the changes of the new contract, which dictates how practices will be paid. You have now learned that part of the new framework has been modified again and processes must be revised once more. What are your options?

　a　You could hold a staff meeting and grumpily inform everyone that there is another change to put in place that won't help the practice or the patients, but will only support the administration level in the health authority. You can then moan for a while about those who have initiated the change and suggest waiting until closer to the deadline for the changes before doing anything.

　Or:

　b　You could hold a meeting and inform staff about the changes, acknowledge that you understand they are feeling weary, but reassure them that this change must happen. You can invite them to look for the positive outcomes of the change, praise them for their hard work so far and schedule a further meeting to create an action group and get started.

What messages does the leader convey in these scenarios?

The leader in (a) shows that moaning, having a negative attitude and delaying taking action are the standards to adopt.

The leader in (b) shows understanding and acknowledgement of the staff's feelings and input and demonstrates a positive attitude and desire for the staff to also adopt that attitude and not delay taking action.

Which of these messages do you think is going to develop staff that perform their jobs with positive attitudes? What kind of atmosphere do you want to create in your business: miserable or upbeat?

2   You are a practice manager new to the surgery and are starting to feel inundated by your workload. You find that regular interruptions from your deputy are taking up large amounts of your time but you continue to smile, stop what you are doing and invite them in, even though you know you'll be staying late to finish your work.

What are your options?

a   You continue to be the 'Nice Boss', working late in the evenings to catch up and becoming more and more tired and stressed. Eventually you snap at your deputy and tell her to stop disturbing you, which has a negative impact on your relationship. She doesn't disturb you as often but now you worry that you might be missing important information.

b   You have a meeting with your assistant and explain that you work best for chunks of time and that you lose your focus even with short interruptions. You explain that the current situation isn't working for you and want to work out a solution that allows you to keep your focus, maintains the relationship and allows her to do her job well. Together you negotiate a new means of communication involving three short meetings a day with each other and agree that if your door is closed it means 'do not disturb'.

What messages does the leader convey in these scenarios?

The leader in (a) shows that they don't know how to address a problem situation and as a result they may 'explode' later on. This can make staff wonder if a problem is simmering underneath, even though the boss looks OK on the outside. This thinking may keep them on edge even when their leader is feeling fine.

The leader in (b) shows that they will calmly discuss problems that arise and seek solutions that work for both parties. It also gives permission and creates the expectation for the assistant to raise problems as they arise rather than keeping them to herself.

What skills and attitudes do you need to lead by example?

1   Self-awareness. This term is associated with the phrase 'emotional intelligence' which was coined by Daniel Goleman.[1] He describes self-awareness as 'the ability to recognise and understand your moods, emotions, and drives, as well as their effect on others'.

2   Self-regulation. This is defined as 'the ability to control or redirect disruptive impulses and moods and the propensity to suspend judgement; to think before acting'.

How do you acquire these skills?

Self-awareness

This is all about what's really going on inside you. How do you feel? What are your thoughts and internal dialogue saying to you? What needs and values are you trying to meet by behaving this way or doing those actions?

Feelings

Sometimes we have a limited vocabulary to describe how we feel, making it harder to pinpoint what's going on inside. The purpose of the list below is to broaden your thinking about your feelings.

Positive feelings which occur when we have our needs and values met:

cheerful	hopeful	enthusiastic	touched
excited	grateful	appreciative	proud
content	optimistic	calm	confident

Negative feelings which occur when our needs and values are not being met:

upset	frustrated	hurt	lonely
impatient	angry	resentful	anxious
worried	frightened	reluctant	guilty

Exercise: Awareness of feelings

To become more aware of your feelings, take a minute at the end of each day and recap how you felt during the day. Look for the words that most accurately describe your feelings. Your increased vocabulary will make your communication clearer when speaking with others as well as helping you empathise with others feelings. Also look for any link between your common feelings and the situations in which they arose. What was happening and what were you thinking?

Values and needs

Values and needs are those things that are really important to us in life and so they are the drivers of our behaviour. When our needs are met, we feel *satisfied*. When our values are met, we feel *fulfilled*. Whether something is a need or a value depends on the intensity of the feeling you experience. For example, one person may *have a need* for a certain level of independence to function adequately, while another, who considers this to be a *value*, is at their most fulfilled and happy when they are independent.

Conversely, when our needs are not being met or our values are not active in our lives, we become dissatisfied, disgruntled and unfulfilled. Something just isn't right, though we may not even know what it is. Identifying and actively bringing your values to life through specific conscious actions, particularly at work, will make you feel a lot more satisfied at the end of the day.

Exercise: Identifying your needs and values

1 Take a few sheets of paper and write your answers in detail to the following questions.

- Think of a time in your professional career when things were going really well for you; picture that time in your mind.
    - What was happening?
    - How did you feel?
- Think of a time in your personal life when things were going really well for you; picture that time in your mind.
    - What was happening?
    - How did you feel?
- Think of a time in your professional career when things were going badly for you; picture that time in your mind.
    - What was happening?
    - What was missing?
    - How did you feel?
- Think of a time in your personal life when things were going badly for you; picture that time in your mind.
    - What was happening?
    - What was missing?
    - How did you feel?
- What really makes you angry? (When something or someone's behaviour conflicts with our values, we often feel angry so this question will give you some more ideas of your values.)

2 Review your answers and write a list of what has come up that is important to you. Think of those things in terms of what you receive and what you give. For example, you may have identified 'support' as being important to you. Is that support from colleagues or giving support to others?

3 Now consider how you feel when you have these things in your life; are you satisfied or fulfilled? Rewrite your list as needs and values.

4 Prioritise your values list by identifying your number one value and then your next top four. (Limit yourself to five core values so you can identify those most essential for you.) To help you decide, ask yourself, 'How would I feel if this were taken from me? How would I feel if I couldn't live like this?'

Here are some further examples of needs and values:

play	variety	relaxation	spontaneity
meaning	purpose	awareness	achievement
learning	growth	beauty	love
nurture	affection	sexual expression	intimacy
protection	security	knowledge	reassurance

to understand	skill	equality	collaboration
honesty	reliability	balance	harmony
autonomy	authenticity	control	empathy
acceptance	to be valued	recognition	celebration
respect	community	belonging	loyalty
support	health	adventure	

There are also fundamental needs such as food/water, warmth and shelter.

5 Add to your existing list any others you have selected from the list above.

6 Once you are aware of your needs and values, you can decide how well they are being met and what you need to introduce more of. Rate how well each need and value is currently being met on a scale of 0–10 where 0 is not being met at all and where 10 is living your values and meeting your needs every day.

7 The next step is to find ways to bring those that scored poorly closer to 10/10. Write your options next to the needs/values you want to improve and select which options you will act upon now. For example to bring celebration into your life, you may suggest to your management team that for 5 minutes each meeting, you share with each other, what is going right in your workplace.

It is usually not practical to have all of your values fulfilled and needs met in the one environment. For example, if you have a need to be loved and accepted (which most people do) it would be most appropriate to have this met in your personal life, rather than in the workplace. However, if one of your values is 'love' then you can behave in a loving manner to your colleagues and staff by being concerned for their well-being and by supporting them.

What you are trying to achieve by identifying your values is whether they are aligned with the values of your workplace. Sometimes it may seem that the government or department of health is not in alignment with what is most important to you. However, this may also be temporary. In this situation, always look at how you can introduce your values into your immediate work environment.

Consider in which other environments you can start living more in line with your values: at home, in a social network, through volunteer work or charities you could support. Think about what living in accordance with your values looks like to you and then try and do more of it within the limits you are presented with. You may only have 10 minutes with a patient but you can still be compassionate.

Ultimately, if your workplace presents a fundamental clash against your values, then it will probably be best for you to find a new employer. Living against your values is soul destroying and therefore best resolved in the interests of your long-term health. Once you are more aware of your feelings and the drivers of your behaviour, you need to acknowledge that your mood, behaviour and actions have an impact on others.

Exercise: The importance of self-awareness

Start consciously noticing the impact that others have. If someone arrives at work in a grumpy mood, notice how that makes you and other people feel and behave. Are they being cautious around that person or has the mood lowered in the department? If the grumpy person is abrupt and rude in the way they speak, what happens to others? Are they rude back?

If you think you couldn't possibly have that effect on other people, test your assumption. The quickest way to find an answer to this is to ask your trusted colleagues and staff: 'What impact do "what I do" and "how I go about it" have on you?' Or instead ask: 'Can you tell if I'm in a bad mood? How does that affect you?'

Also, look at your personal life and see how your partner, wife or children respond to your moods.

Self-regulation

Once you have self-awareness it is important to *act* on it, which is self-regulation. Most importantly, this means controlling impulses and moods that might have a negative impact. However, you can also deliberately adopt a positive mood and perform actions that have a positive impact on others.

Stop reacting, start responding

Sometimes people are in 'react' mode and they express whatever springs to mind without thinking about the consequences. If you can relate to this then a useful exercise for you is to practise 'stepping' into the pause between the stimulus that makes you want to react in a negative way and your response. Use that pause as a thinking space for your self-awareness and self-regulation. To help you remember to go into that space, consider:

- picturing your hand hitting a 'stop' or 'pause' button
- hearing an alarm in your head as an alert that you may say something dangerous or a voice saying 'wait . . .'
- feeling someone's arms holding you still in the pause space.

Emotions

Anger and fear are commonly expressed emotions that can have a negative impact on others. These may present as frustration, rudeness, demands or as panic, among other things. If you experience these feelings *and* express them in a manner detrimental to others, then learning to curb them will be useful.

Exercise: Managing emotions with thoughts

Think of a time at work when you felt angry or afraid. Remember what that felt like and the context of the experience. Slow down that time and consider:

- Where did you feel that emotion in your body? Was it in your stomach, your chest?
- What were you thinking and saying to yourself before that emotion started?

It's best if you can identify the very first thing that happens that then leads to your negative emotions being expressed. This is usually a particular thought. Often people will start catastrophising ('I'm going to get fired for doing this wrongly'), using negative self-talk ('I'm an idiot – how could I have made such a stupid mistake?') or making negative judgements about another person ('They are hopeless at their job – they don't care how this affects the business'). If you are not sure of what that thought process is then notice where you first feel that emotion.

Once you know the thoughts or where the feeling begins in you, use that as a trigger to do something different. Try thinking differently, such as 'Everyone makes mistakes – what can I learn from this' or 'What needs is this person trying to satisfy?'. Think about what thoughts would help you in that situation.

When you first notice the negative feelings, do something different such as a calming exercise of deep breathing, counting slowly backwards from 10 to 0 or by saying 'I need a moment alone'.

Sometimes people handle stressful situations in a manner that seems OK to them but is not perceived to be appropriate by others. For example, some people use humour when they are stressed but this can upset others. Knowing your personality type as discussed in Chapter 4 will also reveal your default behaviour when under stress as well as how it may be perceived. This gives you the opportunity to modify your behaviour according to the situation.

Exercise: Leading by example

1 Decide what impression you want to give and what you want to inspire in others (e.g. positive attitude, self-restraint, punctuality, or courteousness).
2 Think back over the past month and make two lists of what you did to support or detract from that impression. If necessary, ask for input from your colleagues and staff.
3 Looking at your list, highlight what you will continue to do and what you will stop doing.
4 Be more aware of the common situations in which you have trouble self-regulating; these are often situations that seem to push your buttons in a bad way.
5 Commit to pausing and thinking before acting.
6 Recruit friends and co-workers to remind you of your commitment.
7 Evaluate your progress by checking with colleagues how your behaviour has changed after a month.

Suggested learning outcomes and action points

1 Know the definitions of self-awareness and self-regulation.
2 Become more self-aware by exploring your needs and values, your feelings or having a personality-type assessment.
3 Explore how you are currently living according to your values.
4 Explore what needs you have that aren't being met and devise an action plan to get them met.
5 Know how your behaviour changes when you are under stress and have a strategy to modify any behaviour that may be perceived in a negative manner by others.

Reference

1 Goleman D. *Emotional Intelligence: 10th Anniversary Edition; Why It Can Matter More Than IQ.* London: Bantam; 2005.

Further reading

Great leaders of people tend to be politicians, activists, explorers and entrepreneurs so look for their biographies or autobiographies and also books that cite lessons from their experiences. For example:

• Jones S, Gosling J. *Nelson's Way: Leadership Lessons from the Great Commander.* London: Nicholas Brealey Publishing Ltd; 2005.
• Shackleton A, Morrell M, Capparell S. *Shackleton's Way: Leadership Lessons from the Great Antarctic Explorer.* London: Nicholas Brealey Publishing Ltd; 2003.

Chapter 6

Leading by persuasion

When what you say convinces people to follow your lead.

When to use this style

Leading by persuasion involves appealing to people's logic, emotions, values and needs so they are more likely to behave or perform in a manner that will support achievement of the task.

For example, consider two general practices that decide to merge into one new location. As a result, clinical and non-clinical teams will be merged, and systems and standards will be reviewed and updated. This merger is a major change that may be welcomed by some staff but resisted by others. This scenario is ideal for leading by persuasion as you have the opportunity to manage people's fears and expectations and provide reassurance.

In this scenario, those who welcome the changes are seeing opportunities outweighing threats. The merger is appealing because they:

- have the chance to be promoted and earn more money (logic)
- enjoy working in larger teams (emotion)
- see the chance to develop better patient care programmes (values)
- are able to satisfy a need of 'serving/helping others' on a larger scale (needs).

Those who are unhappy about the change may:

- feel threatened that they may lose their job in the restructuring (logic)
- be worried that they won't get along with new team members (emotion)
- believe that the restructuring will create more pressure on them and reduce how well they can do their job (values)
- think they will lose some of the control that they have in their current job which they have a need for (needs).

What skills and attitudes do you need to lead by persuasion?

1 Awareness of other people's emotions, values and needs. If you want to appeal to these elements you must be aware of them in the first place. This awareness begins with consciously listening for and asking about feelings, values and needs.
2 Effective presentation and communication skills. Good presentation skills, whether one-to-one or to groups, allow you to provide a logical argument, acknowledge the challenges of change and encourage a positive view of the situation. You must also have the ability to handle disagreements in response to your argument.

How do you acquire these skills?

Awareness of emotions, values and needs

Emotions are usually fairly easy to read but it's the message they carry that you must look for. If you can't establish at the time what the cause of the emotion is, bear in mind that there may be something else going on in that person's mind, which they are not sharing or perhaps are not even aware of themselves.

For example: someone who is angry may be expressing frustration or hurt at not being involved in making a decision.

To be clear about where an emotion is coming from, guess 'Are you angry because it's important for you to be able to contribute?' or ask 'What made you feel so angry?'. Two notes about this latter question: always ask 'what' instead of 'why' as 'what' is less confrontational. Ask what 'made' them feel a certain way to put those feelings into a past tense instead of perpetuating the negative emotion in the present tense.

If they don't engage in the conversation, share how you are feeling – for example, 'I feel a little frustrated now because I really want to understand what is happening for you at this time. Would you be willing to discuss that?' Give them the opportunity to engage with you, and if they won't, end the meeting, reassuring them that when they want to talk with you, you'll be available.

From Chapter 5, 'Leading by example', you will have an understanding of how your *values and needs* drive your behaviour and influence your emotions. When you want to influence other people it is vital to know what is important to them (i.e. their values and needs).

You can learn this through informal conversations or in a group during a workshop. I like the workshop option because this kind of round-table discussion focuses on topics that really matter to people, allowing sharing and therefore development of trust within the group. This one workshop will help people get to know their workmates better than months of chit-chat. You also have the opportunity to make them more self-aware, to think about how they describe their feelings and needs, and how they in turn drive behaviour. It is important to make this a positive experience. Hence there must be ground rules for maintaining a non-judgemental and objective environment and no tolerance of negative personal comments.

To elicit the values and needs of your staff or colleagues, I recommend that you repeat the 'Identifying your needs and values' exercise from Chapter 5 (p. 42). Questions such as 'What's really important to you?' can be harder to answer and interpret. Often people will say things like money or family, both of which are a means to meet needs. Money may satisfy needs such as 'security' by providing a roof over their head or 'play/adventure' so they can buy a new car. Family may satisfy needs such as 'connection' or 'development/growth'.

Once you have this information and they have more conscious awareness of these things, you can work on how they can bring their values to life more in the workplace. Doing this is relevant to improving joy for staff and the customers, especially in times of change. If possible, show how the result of making changes will allow for staff values and needs to be met even more. If this is not the case, then discuss with staff how they can adhere to their values to maintain good morale while the changes are occurring.

Exercise: Raising your awareness

To increase your awareness of other people's feelings, values and needs, you must practise. Set yourself the daily task of analysing one episode of behaviour. Invest a minute or so thinking, guessing what feelings the person was experiencing and what needs they were trying to meet.

For example, a receptionist appears to be a little abrupt in her tone to a patient. She might be feeling frustrated because she has a pile of letters to type. Speaking to the patient meant she had to stop typing the letters which meant that her need for efficiency was not being met.

Effective presentation and communication skills

First of all, identify how good you are at presenting to a group and at influencing on a one-to-one basis. You can do this by seeking feedback from people that you have worked with in such situations and, of course, from the results that have occurred.

Exercise: What do you do that helps and hinders your influencing ability?

Even if you are good at presenting and influencing, try working with two other colleagues to role-play a situation in which you must influence one of them and have the other person be an observer. Seek specific feedback on your facial expression, arm and hand movements, overall posture, tone and volume of voice and the words you use. Have your observer notice if there are any contradictions between your words and your body language, if your emotions are too intense or not intense enough for the situation, and if you do anything that distracts from your message. You are looking for everything that helps and hinders your ability to influence.

For example, I remember being in a situation where a doctor on a hospital ward was talking with me about a sick family member. All of his communication techniques were very good, but then he started to swing his stethoscope across his chest. It was not only a little distracting but the movement had a carefree feel to it so it removed some of the sincerity and focus he had previously demonstrated. His body language was out of sync with his words.

If you are presenting to a group of people that you already have a trusting relationship with, then the whole process will be much easier. If the relationships are strained because of a lack of trust or respect, then some level of confrontation from the group may be expected.

When presenting your argument there are some points to remember.

1   Begin by thanking everyone for their attendance and appreciating the good work that they do.
2   Agree ground rules with the group to ensure that you all get as much as possible from the meeting. List their answers to 'What could you do to make this meeting

a complete failure?' and 'What could you do to make it a complete success?'. Go through both lists and get people's agreement that they will behave in accordance with the 'success' list and *not* the 'failure' list. Make sure you see *everyone* nodding. If someone isn't nodding, ask them directly if they agree with the rules.

Basic ground rules include:

- being non-judgemental
- being objective and respectful (i.e. focus on ideas not people)
- being succinct (i.e. no waffling)
- letting other people speak without interrupting
- switching mobile phones off
- being punctual (if coming back from breaks).

3   Begin the presentation by explaining the final positive outcome that you have for your proposal.

4   Describe the benefits that are expected in terms of what the individuals, teams, department, patients and business will gain. This uses the traditional selling tool of 'what's in it for me' (WIIFM) as well as appealing to their values, emotions and needs.

5   Ask your staff what business and personal challenges they anticipate will arise as a result of making your proposed changes.

6   Ask your staff how they feel about the changes and what concerns they have. There will need to be some freedom here for expression of emotion but don't let this get out of hand. At the first sign of a personal attack, step in and stop the conversation. Acknowledge the speaker's concerns and refer them back to the ground rules which should have 'keep comments objective and respectful'. Ask them what actions or behaviours they are concerned about and ensure these are objective observations. Do not be blasé!

7   Have a bare-bones strategy for implementing the changes, which shows action points and manages anticipated difficulties. Then invite contribution from everyone else but particularly those who will be affected by or involved in the implementation of this plan.

8   Note their suggestions on how to implement the changes as well as how to manage their concerns, so that you can agree systems for both. For example: staff may feel more involved by receiving the minutes from the meetings of each team (nurses, receptionists, partners). Be sure that the management team's interpretation is accurate; so if the staff say they want to be kept in the loop, ask how they want that to happen. They might be happy with a meeting every two months or they may want a fortnightly progress update.

9   Ensure you finish on a positive, productive note. Check that people understand what they have agreed to do and encourage individuals to be alert to how they can support the process by noticing problems and then working on solutions. Most importantly, finish by agreeing the next meeting date to review progress.

Stage fright

So you know the process to go through, but once you get up in front of a group your knees go weak, your stomach takes up gymnastics and your mind swiftly empties.

Or maybe the basic presentation stuff is OK for you, but you have difficulty handling questions, or attacks, if people try to undermine you.

There are a lot of options available to improve your public speaking ranging from regular Toastmasters[1] meetings to workshops. These are excellent forums in which to practise but here are some basics.

- Practise, practise and practise some more – you have to know what you are talking about to do it with ease.
- Practise with cue cards rather than fully written notes; it's easier to find your place and reduces the temptation to start reading.
- Always practise by speaking out loud, so you can find words that are difficult to say together, and make the appropriate changes.
- Enhance your communication with body language: use appropriate facial expressions and hand movements and move around. Don't wedge your hands in your pockets, jangle keys, pick your nails or anything else distracting.
- Do a test run with some trusted friends so you can get feedback on your body language, tone, anything that distracts from your message.
- Before you start, make sure you are in as comfortable and confident a state as possible. You can do this by deep breathing and then running a movie in your head: seeing yourself presenting brilliantly, seeing and hearing the audience's positive response and seeing the result that you want. There is an exercise to help you enter this state easily in Chapter 7 called 'Anchoring and accessing confidence (p. 55) which I also recommend you do before speaking.
- Prepare yourself for typical, difficult scenarios that may come up. Re-run them in your head and see what emotions they cause in you. If you get angry, think about the emotion you want to feel instead; it may be calm. If you feel terrified, you may want to feel brave or strong instead. You need to develop a tool that instantly brings you in touch with the emotion that you need for those situations. This could be a phrase you say to yourself, taking a deep breath, picturing an image in your head or accessing an anchor (*see* p. 55).
- Once you engage emotions to support you, think about phrases or ways that you will address any attacks. Don't be afraid to interrupt people if they begin to hijack the meeting or forum. Some suggestions are:
  - 'I'm going to have to interrupt you there, John. What I'm hearing from you is that you are unhappy about X. What solutions do you have in mind? . . . Can you have a think about what solutions you believe would be appropriate and bring those to the next meeting please?'
  - 'OK, Jane, thank you. I hear your point and thank you for raising it. We need to move on; who else wanted to make a comment?'
  - 'OK, Jane, thank you. I appreciate your position on this; however, given the overall consensus/the big picture of the situation, my decision is . . .'
  - 'I'm going to have to interrupt you there, John. I understand that this is an emotional topic; however, the purpose of this forum is to identify a strategy for these circumstances, not to air our grievances. This is the situation and we need to find the best possible way to work with it.'
- Don't be afraid of admitting you don't know something. Tell the person you don't know and you'll get back to them or it may be more appropriate to direct them to a resource for the answers they seek.

Suggested learning outcomes and action points

1 Understand what leading by persuasion means.
2 Create an action plan to get to know your colleagues better.
3 Identify how capable you are at presenting to groups and influencing people on a one-to-one basis.
4 Take a presentation skills course or join a Toastmasters group to increase your confidence for group work.
5 Next time you are making a presentation or facilitating a meeting, create ground rules with everyone first and see if this makes a difference.

Reference

1 www.toastmasters.org/

Further reading

- Alder H, Heather B. *NLP in 21 Days: A Complete Introduction and Training Programme*. London: Piatkus Books; 1999.
- Brinkman Dr R, Kirschner Dr R. *Dealing With People you Can't Stand*. New York: McGraw-Hill Publishing Co; 2002.
- Liebling M. *How People Tick: A Guide to Difficult People and How to Handle Them*. London: Kogan Page; 2005.

Chapter 7

Leading by compulsion

Sometimes you just have to tell people what they can and can't do.

When to use this style

Leading by compulsion involves telling people what to do or how to behave and is necessary in several situations. Most obviously, this is appropriate when there is a need to meet a tight time frame such as a medical emergency. It is also valuable when a team is in its early stages of development or when a new staff member begins work. They need to know some basic information that is not debatable and so simply needs to be presented in a direct manner.

Another common situation in which compulsion is needed is when difficult behaviour needs challenging. This behaviour may be coming from patients or other staff. If you are like most people, you are not comfortable with confronting difficult behaviour especially from staff. It is likely that the unacceptable behaviour has continued for some time while you hoped it would just go away.

In dealing with difficult behaviour it is always best to use other styles first, particularly persuasion, as people generally don't like being told what to do. As you practise leading by the other techniques and become more effective at those, you won't need to lead by compulsion as frequently.

Avoiding addressing difficult or inappropriate behaviour is costly in many ways. Consider for a moment that you are a doctor in a partnership and the nurse team leader refuses to participate in the in-house training, which everyone else is required to do.

What are the problems with this?

First, the nurse lead gives a strong signal that for her the in-house training is not important. Because she is in the position to lead by example, the other nurses may follow suit and doubt its importance as well. Second, it shows everyone else in the practice that you don't have to do what the senior management says because she has been allowed to get away with her defiance. If she has been asked repeatedly but still she refuses, it also shows that if you resist for long enough then management will give in. Third, this sends a signal that the management is not a strong, united team as nothing is being formally done.

All of these features may seem fairly innocuous but, when the time comes for more significant changes to occur in the practice, how positively involved do you think this nurse will be, especially if she is not keen on the change? She has already indicated that she doesn't appreciate her role as a team member and that she will defy the requests of the senior management team. This could lead to her other team members refusing to cooperate, despite your best efforts at persuasion.

Alternatively, consider the impact of not confronting a staff member that is rude to another. Let's say Jane has developed a tendency to put Sarah down in front of other staff. This destructive behaviour will most likely continue if not addressed and Sarah may become stressed, take sick leave or retaliate. You may even end up with a bullying complaint in your workplace. Confronting Jane and telling her such behaviour is not acceptable and that she must change her ways involves leading by compulsion. A good leader will aim to understand and resolve what is driving Jane's negative behaviour in order to retain her on staff and bring out her positive attributes.

Dealt with in a fair and objective manner, Jane will know that there are standards she must adhere to and that she has a compassionate boss. The rest of the staff will also learn this lesson and know that the boss is not afraid to do the difficult parts of the job to create a supportive environment for them all.

Are there pitfalls with leading by compulsion? Telling people what to do without seeking their input is also leading by compulsion. If you do this regularly, staff may begin to believe that their opinion doesn't matter and they may feel undervalued.

What skills and attitudes do you need to lead by compulsion?

1 Confidence and courage to lead in an emergency or to tackle difficult situations.
2 Interest in knowing what drives behaviour so you can explore why a particular behaviour has worsened.
3 Non-threatening dialogue to challenge difficult behaviour.
4 Ability to keep the big picture in mind so your goal is to resolve situations while accepting this may result in resignation, patient complaints or simply a period of discomfort while adjustments are made.

How do you acquire these skills?

Confidence and courage

These emotions can be rapidly boosted by reflecting on achievements in your past, particularly those that involved you overcoming fears or uncertainties, or specific situations that turned out better than you expected at the time. You can also access positive emotions from those previous experiences exactly when you need them.

Exercise: Building confidence
- Think of a time when you felt really proud. What were you doing and what was happening?
- Think of a time when you were really brave. What were you doing and what was happening?
- What are the achievements you have had in your life?

When you answer, consider all the different parts of your life including career, learning, social, health and family. Your list may look like this:

- moved to another part of the country and made great friends
- completed my degree
- raised two happy children

- took up running and completed a 10-kilometre race
- decorated my entire apartment
- conquered my fear of flying.

Make your list as long as possible. The more elements you have, the stronger your confidence will be.

Not much on the list?

If you have a short list and none of the elements really give you a strong feeling of confidence, then find something that is a challenge for you. The challenge should make you feel a little nervous when you imagine yourself stepping up to it.

There are all kinds of challenges: physical, emotional, mental and social. For example:

rock climbing	taking further studies with exams
joining a public speaking group	running a race
holding a dinner party	white water rafting
doing volunteer work	

Once you have stepped up to your challenge, you instantly have that to reflect on. Some people wouldn't even step up!

Exercise: Anchoring and accessing confidence

Think of the time that you felt most confident (or calm, courageous, whatever the emotion is that you want to access).

Imagine yourself back in that time and experience what you could see, hear, feel and the positive thoughts that you were having.

Make that experience as rich as possible. Make the image brighter, the feelings stronger, the sounds louder and your thoughts clearer.

As this experience reaches its maximum intensity, press your thumb against your ring finger on the same hand, capturing all of that confidence in one movement. You are anchoring this experience in your mind.

Repeat this a few times and then test it out.

Think of a time that would normally make you feel anxious and then think of it again when pressing your thumb and ring finger together. If you have created a strong anchor, you should feel the positive emotion and a lot less anxiety.

Use this any time that that you need the emotional state that you have captured.

Extra tip

Another strategy is to remind yourself of the positive reason for your actions.

I remember a small-business owner who was faced with having to sack a staff member but felt really uncomfortable with the task. She reminded herself that the staff member's poor performance was reducing the overall income of the business which meant less income for her. She made this more powerful by framing it in her mind as 'this person is taking food off my child's table'. Reminding herself of that gave her the courage and motivation to terminate that person's position.

Remember that every time you lead by compulsion, it becomes easier and further boosts your confidence.

Interest in knowing what drives behaviour

There are many reasons why people behave in a difficult manner and if you can learn what those reasons are, then you can work on specifically targeted solutions.

For example:

- They may be having a personal crisis. A solution may be time off or an adjustment to workload.
- They may be afraid of losing control in some element of their work. Here, reassurance of where they can retain control is needed as well as helping them understand the benefits of relinquishing control.
- They may have low self-esteem and need reassurance that they are doing well and that you have confidence in them. They may need a course to help build their confidence and esteem. Naturally, if you feel that this is best handled by someone with training, then a course, with your reassurance, is the best combination.
- They may be blissfully unaware of how their behaviour is affecting others and need to be told.

Before you talk to the individual involved, gather the facts and get a sense of where the other person is coming from. What are their values and what stressors have occurred in their lives recently? When you then speak with the person, non-threatening dialogue is recommended.

Non-threatening dialogue to challenge difficult behaviour

Dr Marshall Rosenberg[1] describes a four-step process for 'non-violent communication' which is excellent for exploring difficult behaviour. I recommend this technique to address behaviour *as it occurs.* Further steps are added to the process for behaviour that despite your intervention is damaging and unchanging. This is covered in Chapter 15 (p. 136).

The key thing to remember before you begin is be aware that you are exploring, *not* blaming or criticising yourself or the other person involved. You may also want to reassure the person you are talking with that you are looking for solutions and understanding, not blame or criticism, as this is what many people will otherwise be expecting.

The four steps are:

1 observations: these are what you can see or hear – 'When I (see, hear, etc.) . . .'
2 feelings: how you feel in relation to what you are observing – 'I feel . . .'
3 needs: the needs that are creating those feelings 'because I need X/value X/X is really important to me . . .'
4 requests: the concrete actions that you are requesting – 'Would you be willing to . . .'

As an example consider speaking with a staff member who has just yelled at a patient.

1 'When I heard you speak with a raised voice to that patient
2 I felt concerned
3 because being caring is an important value for this practice.
4 Would you be willing to speak in a lower voice?'

(*Note*: State what you want them to do not what you want them to stop doing. Here, you haven't asked them to stop speaking loudly; you've asked them to use a lower voice – a subtle but important difference.)

There is no personal attack in this conversation, only a request, so it is less likely to make the other person defensive.

When you want to understand what has created the other person's behaviour use the first three steps and then ask them: 'Would you be willing to tell me what was happening for you in that situation?'

Again, note the use of the word '*what*' rather than '*why* did you do that?'. This is intentional as people often respond defensively if asked 'why?'. 'What' is perceived as being less threatening and people are more likely to explain their actions rather than defend them.

One of the benefits of this statement is that it is difficult to argue with. You are stating an objective observation and then *your* feelings and needs. Make sure that you keep your feelings and needs related to you. If you hear yourself saying, 'I need *you* to . . .' then your statement becomes a judgement or demand that is likely to make the other person defensive.

Another strategy is the process of 'APISWAPED' by Jonathan Robinson in his book *Communication Miracles for Couples*.[2] It uses similar principles to the non-violent communication techniques with some additions to the beginning and end of the conversation. He uses the following.

Appreciate the person on a regular basis to build your relationship. People feel valued when you appreciate them, and you can do this by giving specific compliments. 'I really appreciated you doing those extra jobs for me today. Otherwise, I would have been running an hour late and feeling stressed. Thank you.'

If most of the time when you speak to people you are asking them to do something for you or correcting them, they will not feel valued or appreciated.

Exercise: Counting compliments

Go through a day listening out for compliments, appreciation and gratitude. Keep score of how many you hear. Then do the same thing for requests or corrections and compare. Aim to have a department or practice where compliments are commonly made.

He also suggests making an appreciative statement at the beginning of this conversation.

Positive intention. This is telling the person what your positive intention is by having the conversation. 'I want to ensure that the whole team is working together as best as possible so I want to talk with you' or 'I want to make sure I'm working as effectively as possible'.

Make sure you keep focused on yourself, not the other person. If you say to them that you want to talk to them to make them understand what they are doing wrong you have instead made a personal attack.

Say what you see is the problem, being objective and not interpreting actions or behaviours. 'I've noticed that you have been arriving late to our meetings' or 'I've noticed that you call me several times a day at my other workplace. This is a problem for me as it breaks my concentration so I end up taking longer to get jobs done.'

Ask person for input and solutions on the problem. 'What is the reason for that? What needs to happen for you to get to the meetings on time? How can I support you? What would be an alternative way of contacting me?'

Give them a chance to speak up but have an idea ready, in case an answer is not forthcoming.

Experimental solution is negotiated. If you have another idea that you want to propose, now is the time. Make sure you come up with a solution that you both think has a good chance of working.

Declare your agreement together to implement the solution and to evaluate the result. 'Let's try that for one week and then have a quick review at 11am on Friday to see how it's working for you.'

Note: be prepared to step into your leadership boots and remind them of your agreement when they slip back into old habits. This will inevitably happen, so create a gentle reminder in their environment from the outset.

For example, if you agree that you are to be contacted by email instead of phone calls, they may like to have a note on their phone that says 'email Dr X' which they will see each time they reach for the phone.

Ability to keep the big picture in mind

Your intention, as the leader, is always to achieve a positive outcome for both parties involved in the negotiation. This may not always be possible.

As the leader you must work at meeting the needs of the task first.

The business has to run effectively to ensure that patient healthcare needs are met. This prime purpose can only be achieved if a multitude of other steps occur, such as having sufficient staff, patient appointments being made with clinicians, staff continuing to develop professionally, clinicians being paid on time, and hygiene being maintained.

The other essential purpose of the business is to create an attractive, supportive environment in which to work. Otherwise there won't be the staff to care for the patients or the staff to support the clinicians who care for patients.

Anything that compromises patient healthcare or the work environment must therefore be addressed as soon as possible. Staff and patients have the ability to affect standards of both these factors and consequently the leader must address both. Strive for commitment from the staff to support the business purposes; however, if they refuse, remove them from the business. Regarding patients this is usually done when they are consistently abusive of staff or the systems that you operate. Always have a fair process to take people through where the last step involves termination of a position, resignation or removal from the practice's patient list.

The greatest challenge among people who dislike taking disciplinary action is their need to protect and care for others. In those disciplinary situations they strongly feel that they are doing the exact opposite to the individual in front of them. Accordingly, they find reasons to keep them on and to give another chance, despite the fair process they have been through, which has been unsuccessful.

If you find yourself in this situation, shift your focus to protecting and caring for the customers/patients, the other staff members, the organisation as a workplace and yourself rather than focus on one individual. Think also of the negative consequences of keeping those who are not performing (i.e. patient ill health, good staff leaving and potential litigation) and you will probably find the strength to go through with the process as described.

Suggested learning outcomes and action points

1 Understand why you must have the skills to lead by compulsion as it will inevitably be necessary.
2 Be able to identify situations where leading by compulsion is necessary and advantageous.
3 If leading by compulsion makes you uncomfortable, identify exactly what the obstacles are for you to use this technique.
4 Seek mentoring or coaching so you are able to use this technique without being stressed by it.

References

1 Rosenberg M. *Nonviolent Communication: A Language of Life: Create Your Life, Your Relation-ships and Your World in Harmony with Your Values*. Encinitas, USA: PuddleDancer Press; 2003. (www.CNVC.org and www.NonviolentCommunication.com)
2 Robinson J. *Communication Miracles for Couples: Easy and Effective Tools to Create More Love and Less Conflict*. Berkeley, USA: Conari Press; 1997.

Chapter 8

Leading by enabling with coaching, training and support

Finding the most effective way to develop people and their skills.

When to use this style

Coaching, training and support are suited to learning situations and therefore it is worth bearing in mind the experiments of Robert Rosenthal mentioned in Chapter 1. These demonstrated the impact of teacher's expectations on the performance of their students. The group 'labelled' as more intelligent out-performed the group 'labelled' less intelligent. As a general rule, people will live up *or* down to the labels given to them. The label becomes a self-fulfilling prophecy.

Moreover, the influences on how people decide their labels can be overt or covert. Imagine how you would feel joining a team called the 'Alpha Group', 'Super Staff' or the 'Genius Group' compared with a team called the 'Losers', 'Dim-Wits' or 'Good-for-Nothings'. Now these are glaring, overt labels but you will have felt in yourself the groups you'd rather be a part of and which ones would inspire you to perform better.

A person may not actually say something aloud, but a message may get through covertly with

- the silent treatment
- indifference
- not having challenging tasks from the boss or colleagues
- the boss solving problems on their own without seeking your input.

Be aware that being helpful and solving problems independently or being quiet and letting someone get on with their job may be interpreted in a negative way by your staff. It is crucial to communicate your positive feelings and compliments effectively so people really do know that you are labelling them in a positive way. Similarly, stepping back from being the 'fix-it' person will not only show your trust in others, but allow them to develop and get further positive feedback.

The difference between coaching, training and support

Coaching is a non-directive way of developing knowledge and learning as it relies on drawing ideas and suggestions from the individual or group. There are benefits for all parties from using this process including greater commitment to ideas and hence greater likelihood of action to be taken, stimulating creative, independent thinking, increased confidence in their own resourcefulness, less perception of you as the easy option to get a problem solved and hence less demands on your time.

Training is a directive way of developing knowledge and learning and is most appropriate for teaching standard systems or techniques and new concepts. For example, training would be appropriate when teaching a new member of the team how the computer system works.

Support occurs on two levels. On a situational level you ensure that the learner knows you are available to provide tangible resources as well as be active in their development or achievement of a task. For example, if a staff member refuses to help the learner or deliberately sabotages their progress, then as the leader you would step in to address the unhelpful staff member's behaviour. The other level of support is an intellectual and emotional one in which you positively 'label' them, and convey that you have confidence in them.

When do I coach, train or support?

Often a combination of these styles will create the best learning experience for an individual but here is a general guide.

Support is needed for people feeling overwhelmed, uncertain or lacking in confidence, no matter what their skill level is. Particularly look out for this in people who have a high skill level and may not be comfortable admitting these uncertainties. As you offer support, be certain of how it is interpreted by the other person; do they think you don't believe in their capability or do they simply see the offer as support when they need and request it?

Training and coaching are often used in combination, but as a general rule, the greater the person's skill level in a particular field, the more coaching should be done when working on that field of expertise. Try to use as much coaching as possible as it provides a more stimulating learning experience. The time not to use coaching is when someone is feeling overwhelmed, like they are moving in circles or are up against a brick wall. Giving them useful suggestions helps break them out of overwhelm mode and shows your support as a resource when they really need you.

For example: a medical student is learning how to break bad news to a patient.

As their trainer if you are in directive training mode you will say: 'I'd say . . .' or 'Tell them . . .' or 'This is the recommended way . . .'.

If you are in non-directive coaching mode you will say: 'What do you think would be the most appropriate way to do this? What do you think they might be feeling? How might you help them with those feelings? What else do you want to think about in terms of how you'll use your body language and the environment?'

Obviously being non-directive will take longer. However, the experience and result usually remains in the learner's mind so you won't have to repeat yourself when the same situation comes up again.

The importance of evaluation

When taking on a new recruit, you will hopefully have predetermined that they are capable of doing the fundamentals of the job. On the job observation, seeking feedback from colleagues and feedback from the individual should be undertaken in a non-threatening manner with a view to support the person as much as necessary.

In addition to job skills, staff need to learn the operating procedures and culture of an organisation. Operating procedures describe how to send referrals, how to get paid or how a patient is registered with a practice.

Culture involves learning the expectations and standards regarding behaviour such as leadership, participation as a team member, awareness of areas for improvement, sense of fun while working or innovation for problem solving.

Training has a role in highlighting systems that support a culture. For example, the monthly meeting has 10 minutes for raising areas for improvement and solutions and 10 minutes for acknowledging mistakes and successes. Coaching supports the learning of culture by encouraging people to think in new ways, to have the confidence to contribute and to be innovative in their actions.

What skills and attitudes do you need to lead by enabling with coaching, training and support?

1　Coaching skills.
2　Training requires flexibility to adapt delivery to the individual's needs. You need to have written operating procedures, be able to demonstrate techniques/skills, and have a means of measuring performance.
3　Effective feedback.
4　Patience and willingness to invest time to develop people and to challenge those who do not support development.

How do you acquire these skills?

Coaching skills

These allow you to ask the questions and make observations that allow the coachee (person being coached) to come up with their own answers and decide what is the best solution or course of action. Purists will say that you must *not* give suggestions or ideas to the coachee; however, as already mentioned, this is necessary in some situations.

For an introduction to coaching techniques there are a range of good books including:

- *Effective Coaching* by Myles Downey[1]
- *Coaching for Performance* by John Whitmore[2]
- *The Manager as Coach* by Eric Parsloe[3]
- *Coaching and Mentoring in Health and Social Care* by Julia Foster-Turner.[4]

Coaching courses are available through universities, personnel organisations such as the Chartered Institute of Personnel Development (www.cipd.co.uk) and private coach training organisations. Some courses represent a joint venture between business schools and private institutions. Courses are constantly being updated and changed so I recommend that you do your own research and speak with people who have completed their training with the institution you are considering.

Importantly, national occupational standards for coaching qualifications are being developed by ENTO which is a UK Standard Setting Body. See www.ento. co.uk for the latest update. Particularly bear these standards in mind when choosing a course from a private institution.

Fundamental skills

The fundamental skills required to coach are effective questioning and listening without judgement. Some coaches also use a formula (such as the GROW model which stands for Goal, Reality, Options and Will and Way forward) for a coaching session to ensure outcomes are reached. Additionally, when the coach has the expectation that the client is extremely resourceful, it allows the coach to wait and give the client time to think of their own answers.

Effective questioning

Use it:

- to help people think beyond obstacles. Ask them to think of the goal they want or the 'what' instead of the 'how' (e.g. 'What is our goal/the end result we are trying to achieve? If you had unlimited resources what would you aim for? If you had enormous confidence what could you achieve?').
- to brainstorm a lot of ideas. Continue to ask 'and what else could you do/the team do/the organisation do?'.
- to encourage action and ownership of ideas. Ask: 'From that list of options [which they created], which one looks the most appealing to do? Which one would have the biggest impact on achieving your goal? Which one will you do?'
- to see a situation from different points of view. 'If you imagine yourself in the patient's/other person's position, what might they be experiencing? If you imagine yourself as a fly on the wall observing that interaction, what do you see contributing to the problem? What is helping?'
- to challenge limiting beliefs and behaviours such as if a person says they are 'hopeless' at their work. Ask 'What makes you think that? Do you think you're hopeless at *everything* about your work?' Usually they will say, 'Well, not everything' so you can then refocus them on what they are good at with 'I know you are great at X and the other staff think you are brilliant at Y; what else are you good at?'

Obstacles to effective questioning:

- Offering answers instead of allowing the person the opportunity to come up with their own.
- Jumping into the silence to ask another question; this silence is usually when the person is thinking.

Solutions:

- To stop yourself jumping in on the person's silence; think 'WAIT or Why Am I Talking?'

- Have a pre-prepared list of a few favourite questions designed to achieve different outcomes. Once you have listened to the coachee, you can ask for a moment to think yourself, and check your list.
- Tell the other person you will wait for them to speak so they can expect the silences.

Effective listening

Often when we think we are listening, we are not. We may not even be hearing what the person is saying and instead are creating one or more obstacles (*see* below). Even if we do hear the person's words we may not be picking up the deeper elements of the communication – for example, when someone says they are going to take a particular action but their tone and level of enthusiasm suggest they are afraid or hesitant to do what they've just said. When you hear those deeper elements you can use effective questioning to explore them further. If these are not addressed, it is unlikely that the person will actually do what they have said. Obstacles to effective listening:

- Thinking about what you are going to say next.
- Recalling a similar experience you have had.
- Making a judgement of the person talking or the situation they are talking about.
- Day dreaming/wondering what you will have for dinner.
- Trying to think up a solution to the person's problem.
- Hoping the other person will stop talking so you can talk instead.

Solutions:

- Be aware of what is going on in your head. If you find yourself creating any of these obstacles, just refocus on what the person is saying.
- If you find that you tend to make judgements about particular types of people or their behaviour, you may seek some coaching yourself to overcome that or, ultimately, decide you can't work with them.
- Get into the habit of asking people to repeat themselves if you drift off – for example; 'Could you please repeat what you just said? I want to give that more attention.'
- Try a visualisation technique like imagining a pair of antennae on your head so you are extra-sensitive to the unspoken communication.

The formula – the GROW model

This formula can be applied to goals which need to be completed in 10 years or 10 minutes. When you are working on a long-term goal, you keep applying this formula to each step in the strategy until you achieve tangible action points.

Goal

This is identifying the goal for the conversation or for months ahead.

Ask: 'What do you want to get out of this conversation?' or 'What do you want to achieve related to X?' or 'What would need to happen in the next three months related to X for you to feel really proud?'

Reality
This is a statement of where the person is right now, in relation to their goal.

If you are using this process to create strategy, action points and accountability for reaching a goal then the process is quite straightforward.

Ask: 'So what's the current situation compared to that goal?'

If you are using this process for problem solving, this is also the opportunity to explore the background to their issues.

Ask: 'What do you think is getting in the way/could get in the way of you achieving that goal?' or ask the YOW question: 'What role do you think You, Other people and the Workplace (culture, physical layout, physical environment, equipment) are playing in this issue?'

Options
This involves brainstorming as many options as possible to help to achieve the goal.

If this process is for problem solving then consider options in relation to the YOW answers as this is where you will find a broad range of long-term solutions.

To expand options use the traffic-light approach.

Ask: 'What do you need to *start* doing, *stop* doing and *continue* doing to reach your goal?'

Will and way forward
The person now selects which option(s) to put into action.

Ask: 'Which option is the most appealing for you?' and 'Which option would give you the biggest leap toward reaching your goal?'

Then assess their willingness to actually do it.

Ask: 'Rate on a scale of 0–10 (where 0 is no chance and 10 is an absolute certainty) how likely you are to do the action you have chosen.'

As a general rule if they answer less than 8, it's not going to happen.

Ask: 'What do you need to make that a 9/10?'

This opens up the opportunity to explore what extra support they may need or how to minimise the risks associated with a particular option.

Once you have been using the GROW model for a while you will find it easier to move between the four elements during the one conversation instead of feeling the need to use the model in a linear fashion. This allows for a smoother-flowing conversation.

Training

Training means delivering information in a manner that is *easiest for the learner* to receive and assimilate, so you must be flexible. It is also useful to remind yourself of the different learning styles (visual, auditory, tactile/kinaesthetic, active, reflective, sequential and global) from Chapter 4.

Try to identify the person's preferred styles in the beginning so the teaching and learning is easier. Ask them directly, 'How do you prefer to learn?' If they are not sure, then ask any of these questions:

- Would you like to take notes?
- Would a diagram be helpful?

- Shall I tell you how this is done?
- Do you want to have a go at doing this yourself?
- Do you want me to give you the big picture first or the details?

Usually once you start questioning people they'll tell you whether or not they like your suggestions. If they can only tell you what they don't like, then write that down and check what the opposite is; this should reveal their learning style.

Note: it is uncommon for people to learn a new task or behaviour after one training/learning session so expect to repeat the training or coaching several times until the level of performance required is reached.

Effective feedback

There are some key features of giving feedback which make the information more effective.

Dos

- Be objective. State observed actions and the results of them (e.g. 'After you spoke with a raised voice to the patient they became aggressive').
- Be clear about what you want to say and the result you want (i.e. do you want to boost confidence through a compliment, get an explanation from someone about their behaviour or actions, or make the person aware of an error they've made).
- Give positive feedback regularly. Try and catch your colleagues, boss or direct reports doing a good job and compliment them. This allows you to build a positive, trusting relationship with other staff so your first conversation with them is not about what they are doing wrong or what they need to improve
- Give feedback at an appropriate time. This is not a once-a-year event when you do an appraisal. Ideally, give feedback as soon as possible in 'real time'.
- If you need to address *negative behaviour* by a staff member or patient, do it immediately. If it is an emotionally charged event, you may wish to explore the reasons for the problem at a more appropriate time. Don't leave it so long that the incident is half forgotten.
- If you want to give *positive feedback* it is not critical to do it immediately, and you may wish to wait for a lunch break or quiet moment. (*Note*: If you generally don't have any time in your day to do this, then ensure that there is a 'positive feedback' item on the staff meeting agenda. You also need to review how you use your time because without this small amount of freedom in your day you will have no time to be a successful leader.)
- Be honest, respectful and sensitive to how your information will impact the receiver.

Don'ts

- Don't cast judgement or presume you know what someone is thinking (e.g. 'You don't care about your job').

- Don't overly delay giving feedback that will enhance someone's ability to do their job whether that is by building their confidence or correcting their mistakes. Bear in mind: 'feedback delayed is feedback denied'.

Special note

Sometimes people become embarrassed when they are given positive feedback, so they deny or belittle their abilities. They may say they were lucky or it was a one-off event. The problem with this attitude is that the person doesn't attribute a positive result to their internal skills, talents or characteristics. The result of this can be low self-confidence or self-esteem, which may impact on many areas of life such as coping with feedback to address poor performance, dealing with difficult behaviour or taking on new tasks and roles. For this reason it is worthwhile encouraging people to accept compliments.

So how do you handle this?

It's important to make sure the person does receive your positive feedback. You can achieve this by requesting that they accept your compliment or feedback because showing gratitude is important to you.

Then pause so they can do as you've asked (which they undoubtedly will) and thank them.

Move swiftly on at this point so there are no painful silences or further embarrassment.

> Sarah: 'Jo, I really appreciate that you always have a smile ready in the morning. It gives me a little boost of joy for my day. Thank you.'
> Jo: 'Oh, it's nothing. Don't be silly.'
> Sarah: Well, it means a lot to me and it's important to me to show my gratitude, so could you just say ''you're welcome''?'
> Jo: 'Of course, you're welcome.'
> Sarah: 'Thanks.'

Patience and willingness to invest time in developing people

Become aware of how you feel when you are delivering training, coaching or supporting people. If you notice that you feel impatient, this is usually because you are not having your information received as you expect or would prefer. This may be because the person doesn't understand or may be trying to correct the information you are giving them.

For both situations you need to calm yourself first. Do this by:

- taking a quiet, deep breath or counting to five in your head
- calling a 'time out' for a drink or a comfort break so you can change environment and leave the area of tension for a few minutes.

If the person doesn't understand the information you are giving:

- ask for help by asking the learner if you are being clear; ask what they want you to explain in more detail; ask what they want you to repeat or describe in a different way

- use metaphors or stories to describe scenarios
- make sure you have used all three strategies of 'telling, showing' and allowing them to 'do' a new task or behaviour
- ask them to repeat back to you what they have just heard, so you can check understanding.

If the person is correcting the information and coming across as a 'know-it-all':

- suggest that they follow the current procedures for a couple of weeks and to then give you feedback on what they think can be improved; explain the process for suggesting improvements that you have in your department or practice
- thank them for their input and state that you will consider/review what they have said; remember they might be right or have a great idea.

To increase your willingness to deliver training, coaching and giving support, think of all the benefits you and your department will gain, such as strong relationships among staff, greater engagement in work, higher skill levels, innovation and more time. This leadership style facilitates having capable people to delegate to and staff with a greater sense of responsibility. Also consider the opposite: you doing most of the work on your own because there is no-one else to delegate to, people bringing all the problems to you for fixing, feeling constantly pressed for time, working long hours and generally being very stressed. Which would you prefer?

Suggested learning outcomes and action points

1 Understand the difference between coaching and training, particularly directed or non-directed learning.
2 Practise effective listening. Identify a conversation in which you will be aware whether or not you are *really* listening to the other person.
3 Practise effective questioning. Write a short list of problem-solving questions to ask instead of offering a solution immediately.
4 Hold a conversation or run a meeting using the GROW model.
5 Practise giving feedback and set a goal of giving positive feedback to each colleague at least once a week.

References

1 Downey M. *Effective Coaching*. London: Texere; 2001.
2 Whitmore J. *Coaching for Performance*. London: Nicholas Brealey Publishing; 2002.
3 Parsloe E. *The Manager as Coach*. London: Chartered Institute of Personnel and Development; 2001.
4 Foster-Turner J. *Coaching and Mentoring in Health and Social Care*. Oxford: Radcliffe Publishing; 2005.

Further reading

- Whitworth L, Kimsey-House H, Sandahl P. *Co-Active Coaching*. Palo Alto, USA: Davies-Black Publishing; 1998.

Chapter 9

Leading by enabling with trust

Letting go of control to allow other people to have a go.

When to use this style

Leading by enabling with trust gives people freedom and boosts their confidence to do a job. You give them the support with your belief that they can and will perform to, and even exceed, the expected standard. You trust them to do the job properly in clinical and/or business situations. This type of leadership can be particularly difficult for leaders who feel a strong need for control.

Consider teaching a medical student how to excise a mole, or a colleague how to run a meeting effectively or having your reception team leader create a new patient admission system. Telling them 'I believe you can do it' during their preparation for a new activity may be the difference between them having confidence to succeed and achieving a less successful result due to nervousness.

A word of warning: it is vital that your belief in an individual or team and their capability is formed from evidence. Acting on an unfounded belief and encouraging a person or team to do a task that they truly are not capable of is setting them up for a painful failure.

Your evidence can comprise skills or attributes that:

- you have observed directly
- colleagues have reported
- the individual has used or developed in other unrelated situations, particularly in their personal life (e.g. 'As a mum you've taken on a lot of different roles successfully, so you have the ability to handle more than one role, which you can apply to this new job').

Having this evidence is valuable to present to the person who you are supporting, especially if they ask: 'Why do you believe I can do it?'

What skills and attitudes do you need to lead by enabling with trust?

1 Trust in others.
2 Ability to let others work independently and let go of control.
3 Belief that 'there is no failure, only learning'.

How do you acquire these skills?

Trust in others

This step depends largely on you. Do you believe that trust is earned or that you can or must instantly trust others?

Consider a scenario where your colleague is learning to run a meeting effectively. You're not really sure if they can do this but you say 'You'll be fine; of course you can do it'. You might be saying this to be kind or to avoid having to do the training but the end result is poor. The meeting runs over time; your colleague is nervous and moves between talking excessively and not having the courage to keep other speakers succinct. The agenda isn't completed, no action points come from the meeting and everyone leaves feeling that it was a waste of time. The attendees of the meeting also know that you are the one responsible for training your colleague in this new skill.

What are the possible consequences?

- Your colleague feels the pain of a stressful and unsuccessful experience (they are embarrassed and their confidence drops).
- Your colleague's trust in you reduces greatly and they now don't believe what you say.
- You lose credibility as a trainer or mentor in the eyes of those who attended the meeting.
- You must invest large amounts of time rebuilding the relationship with your colleague and your credibility as a trainer.

Because these consequences can take a long time to recover from (i.e. damaged confidence and reputation), I recommend that you find evidence before declaring your trust.

It doesn't have to take a long time to develop this trust, just a keenness to find evidence on which to build the trust. Get to know the person through informal chats about their home life, hobbies, and previous challenges at work as well as asking their colleagues what that person is doing well.

You don't necessarily need to ask about what they could improve, as giving work that plays to people's strengths is rewarding for them as well as for your bottom line and environment.

Ability to let others work independently and let go of control

A lot of people have difficulty with letting go of control. Think of the mum who is pressed for time but will still do all the housework even if her husband offers to help because 'he doesn't do it properly'. It's the same scenario for the doctor who won't delegate administrative tasks because they want to check that everything's correct.

The key question here is: 'What needs to happen for you to be comfortable with someone else doing this particular job?''

The answers to this question will give you a checklist of steps the other person can meet, which will help with making you comfortable with relinquishing your control. As you continue to do this, you will find you won't have to spell out the detail as much. You will find it easier telling them the end result you want and then allowing them to achieve it in the way they think is best.

When you are delegating tasks and letting go of control, it is important for you to explain to people why you are providing details on how to complete a task. Otherwise, it could be perceived by these people as a lack of trust or belief in them.

For example, 'I'm trying to improve my delegating and letting go of control. In the past I've had real trouble with this, so I'd like you to bear with me, until I get the hang of it. For me to feel comfortable with delegating, I would like you to do the job by following these pointers. As we work together, and I'm happy with the standard and the way that we work together, then I'll be more comfortable with letting you just get on with it. Is that OK?'

A scenario example

You are a solo general practitioner who has been doing it all: running the business and seeing the patients. You have just taken on a part-time practice manager and you want to have some building work done to expand your premises. You know it's logical to have the practice manager source builders and architects but you are reluctant to put this project into someone else's hands.

'What do you need to happen to be comfortable with your practice manager doing this job?'

You might want to specify that:

- the practice manager gets quotes from at least three architects and three builders (preferably word-of-mouth referrals)
- the practice manager gets references from past clients of the builders and architects and interviews them with regard to their standard of service, standard of building, ease of working with them, their flexibility for any changes and their ability to deliver the job on time
- once the list of potential providers is narrowed, the practice manager makes an on-site visit to previous jobs to review the completed product
- a half-hour meeting once a week is arranged with the practice manager to discuss findings, progress and problems
- a reasonable time-line has been agreed in which to have these steps completed.

Delegation

Stephen Covey, in his book *The Seven Habits of Highly Effective People*,[1] discusses two types of delegation, which result in two ways you can treat the people you are delegating to.

'Gofer' delegation occurs when you tell people to 'go for this, go for that, do this, do that and tell me when it's done'. You remain responsible for the end result and tell the person everything required, particularly how to do the task. These people are simply *doing* the job. It is extremely hard to give up the control of how a task is done when you are ultimately responsible, but when you can, you move into 'stewardship' delegation.

'Stewardship' delegation focuses on the results instead of the methods. The steward (not you) is responsible for the methods they use and the result that they achieve. They have responsibility for how it gets done and should therefore have greater input into the time frame for the job's completion as they may be more aware of the steps involved. These people *own* the job.

Your role when delegating is to:

- advise of the required end result or the purpose of the task

- provide the deadline for the task if necessary, or agree a time-line together
- ensure the necessary resources are available at the beginning and during the project
- give them advice on what not to do if you know there are certain traps they are likely to encounter; don't tell them what to do as you start to make them a 'gofer' again
- advise them on your availability for support and guidance
- discuss the consequences of task achievement or otherwise in terms of job assignments, rewards, etc.; if this is an assignment to see how well the person can handle a particular type of project for future cases, inform them so they are fully aware of the context
- seek their commitment to the work
- ensure they know your belief in them.

As you surround yourself with capable stewards, you will become more and more comfortable with delegation and letting go of control.

A note on being a perfectionist

Some tasks need perfectionism as a standard. You can't have a cardio-thoracic surgeon performing a coronary artery bypass graft operation and saying, 'Well, most of those stitches are holding the graft in place and it's leaking a bit of blood, but that'll do.' However, perfectionism can be a hindrance when that high standard is not necessary and the costs of producing work to that standard outweigh the benefits.

What is your perfectionism costing you?

Are you missing deadlines for projects or assignments? Are you spending so much time on these tasks that you have less time for your family and no time for you? Are you driving your work colleagues crazy with unnecessary inflated standards?

The key word here is 'unnecessary'. You are producing work to a standard that is very high but doing so comes at a cost. So how do you become more comfortable with not reaching such perfection levels? Well if the words in your head are 'low standard', 'poor quality', 'less than perfect' or 'minimum' then you are not going to change your standards. Having worked with perfectionists, I know it is vital that you use language that doesn't have negative connotations. Think of producing work to the 'required', 'accepted', 'desired' or 'necessary' standard instead and get into the habit of establishing what that level is before you start the job, so you don't waste precious time.

Once you submit work of the 'required' standard, you will have more time to be a perfectionist in other more necessary areas. Additionally, the freedom you experience from this may transfer to other parts of your life allowing you to give up the idea of being 'perfect'.

Belief that 'there is no failure, only learning'

If people believe that making a mistake at work will result in punishment then they will quickly adopt a 'play it safe' approach. They will not want to try out new roles and responsibilities and their creativity and innovation will be tempered. Even more worrying is that they may try to hide a mistake they have made, clinical or otherwise.

However, this belief does not mean that if people make errors in the fundamental components of jobs, their performance should not be addressed. If people are not performing to the expected standard then discussions on root causes need to take place.

What you are aiming to stimulate in people when you say 'there are no mistakes, just opportunities for learning' is a scientist's approach. That means coming up with creative and innovative ideas on how to achieve a desired result. It also means that if one of these ideas doesn't work it is not a failure; it is a chance to examine the detail and ask:

- 'Which parts of this idea that worked are worth keeping?'
- 'Which parts didn't work and can be let go?'
- 'What obstacles arose that prevented a successful result?'
- 'What can we learn from this experience?'

Creating a learning culture

To ensure that all staff appreciate the department or practice philosophy, you must practise what you preach. If errors occur in the workplace, look for problems in the systems that were involved rather than seeking to blame an individual or find a scapegoat.

Tips for creating a learning culture

1   Set a new standard that every staff member brings along at least one idea for business development, team development or patient care improvement every month. Ensure that contributions are recorded in the minutes of the meeting as well as how many ideas are contributed per person, per month. Generally, if people aren't offering ideas it is because they don't believe there is a fair process to evaluate them, they don't believe their thoughts are valuable or they don't believe that management is really interested and they are being paid lip service only, or they might just prefer not to contribute all the time, particularly if someone else has come up with an idea. This is an opportunity to practise enabling others and involving them in creation of the evaluation process.

    At these meetings, present information and feedback from those that your practice serves (i.e. patients, the primary care trust and other general practices). This reinforces that the business develops by learning from all of its customers.

2   Have part of the regular staff meeting dedicated to presenting ideas, celebrating successes and learning from mistakes. This will encourage creativity, problem solving (not problem presenting), engagement and responsibility.

    When there are a large number of staff in multiple teams, meeting with everyone may not be practical. It is more reasonable then to have individual team meetings that go through this process. The group can then select their top ideas to suggest for trial, or implementation to a core group. This core group would comprise key people, such as the team leaders, business owners and managers who then evaluate and agree ideas with which to go ahead. These decisions should be fed back to all contributors through the meeting minutes.

Suggested learning outcomes and action points

1 Recognise the negative effects of your unwillingness to give up control, on others and yourself.
2 Understand the differences between 'gofer' and 'stewardship' delegation.
3 Think of a job that you would like to delegate, select a good steward and set a date and time to meet with them.
4 Identify any issues that you have with letting go of control and seek mentoring or coaching to address those.
5 Co-create an action plan with your staff to instil a learning culture in your business/department.

Reference

• Covey S. *The Seven Habits of Highly Effective People*. 1st ed. New York: Simon & Schuster; 1990.

Chapter 10

Five steps to become a better leader

A step-by-step guide for individuals

So far, you have learned Adair's action-centred leadership model, which can be applied to any leadership situation. You also know five styles of leadership, their associated skills and attitudes, and how to match situations to styles. This chapter gives you a process to implement what you have learned so far.

Before you begin this process there are some key attitudes to adopt to make it easier.

Say these out loud:

- This is all a learning experience.
- I take feedback objectively, not personally.
- I am responsible for making changes.
- This process takes time and I must be patient with myself and others.

Without adopting these attitudes, you may take feedback personally, see a lot of it as criticism and feel like the whole process is taking too long.

The five-step 'ISAGOAL' process

1 Informing others.
2 Self-Awareness.
3 Goal setting.
4 Options for action.
5 Act and Learn.

Step 1: Informing others

As you develop into a greater leader you will need input from your colleagues and staff to raise your awareness, monitor your progress and give you support.

If you already have good relationships then this step involves asking for their:

- feedback formally, now, six and 12 months later as you monitor your progress; on-the-spot feedback during your day-to-day interactions is also valuable
- patience as you make changes
- support/involvement in correcting any negative, former behaviours and in introducing new positive ones.

If your relationships are neutral or maybe even poor, then you must consider further preparatory steps before moving on.

In this respect, there are two excellent communication techniques for repairing neutral or poor relationships. Mixing elements of the Apology framework (AAAR)

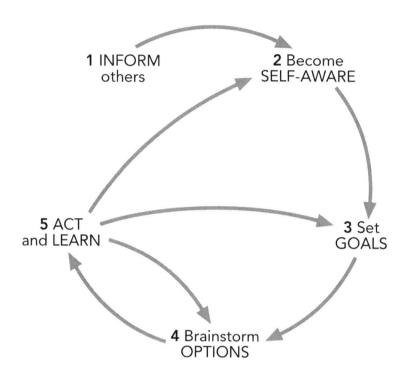

Figure 10.1 The ISAGOAL process.

and APISWAPED by Jonathan Robinson[1] (*see* Chapter 7, p. 57, for more detail) will give you a framework for a dialogue that should be well received even by the most cynical and negative person. Remember that these are just the words involved and you will convey even more through the authenticity and sincerity in your tone, volume and body language.

AAAR – Apology framework

- **Acknowledge** your actions.
- **Apologise** by saying 'I apologise' rather than 'I'm sorry' (which suggests you are a sorry person).
- Make **Amends** by asking 'What can I do to make amends?'
- **Re-commit** to the relationship declaring 'Our relationship is very important; I want you to know I am committed to that.'

APISWAPED

- **Appreciate** the person on a regular basis to build your relationship. Do this by telling them specifically what you appreciate or admire about them.

- **Positive Intention**. This is telling the person what your positive intention is by having this conversation.
- **Say What** you see is the problem, remembering to be objective and not interpreting actions or behaviours.
- **Ask Person** for input and solutions on the problem.
- **Experimental** solution is negotiated, at which point you may need to suggest your solutions.
- **Declare** your agreement to perform the solution and to evaluate the result.

Example

I acknowledge that I haven't always given you the direction/opportunities/support that you've wanted and I apologise. (Acknowledge. Apologise.)

I appreciate that you are all very good at your jobs and have a lot of valuable input and ideas on how we can work better together. (Appreciate.)

This is what I want to achieve: a more positive, efficient workplace where we are all getting our jobs done, enjoying the work and enjoying each other's company. (Positive intention.)

What I'm going to be doing to improve how well I work and how I support you is leadership development. (Offer your solution.)

What I need from you is your:

- feedback now and over the coming 12 months
- patience as I make changes
- support/involvement in correcting any negative, old behaviours and in introducing new ones.

Do you have any other suggestions on how you might like to help me? (Ask person.)

So, we are agreed that I will be doing (action) . . . and you will (action) . . . (Seek and declare agreement.)

Step 2: Self-awareness

Becoming more self-aware through assessments gives you a baseline against which to measure your progress and, most importantly, specific points on which you can take action. You can do this with a self-assessment. Feedback from those you interact with on a regular basis will, however, often give you greater insight. One of the most effective methods of gathering information from others is via 360° feedback. Remember, being a leader means that others will follow you, so you need to see yourself from their point of view. *See* Table 10.1.

Table 10.1 Self-assessment questionnaire: leadership functions and features.
Tick the box with your answer.

Functions	Good at	Need to do more	Need to do less
Planning			
Seeking all available information from the relevant people			
Defining group task, purpose or goal			
Making a workable plan in conjunction with the relevant people			
Initiating			
Briefing the group on the purpose and the plan			
Explaining why the goal or plan is necessary			
Allocating tasks to group members (utilising their strengths where possible)			
Setting/eliciting group standards (for behaviour, performance and achievement steps)			
Controlling			
Maintaining group standards			
Influencing tempo (creating urgency or calming action)			
Ensuring all actions are taken towards objectives			
Keeping discussion relevant			
Prodding the group to action/decision			
Making the final decision when necessary (e.g. when no consensus is reached despite rigorous debate)			
Supporting			
Expressing acceptance of people and their contribution			
Encouraging the team and individuals			
Disciplining the team and individuals (as needed to maintain standards and progress)			
Creating/stimulating team spirit, sense of purpose and accountability			
Reconciling disagreements or encouraging others to explore them			

Functions	Good at	Need to do more	Need to do less
Informing			
Clarifying the task and plan once it has been initiated			
Providing new information to the group so they are aware of the big picture			
Receiving information from the group so you are able to monitor progress			
Summarising suggestions and ideas coherently so that you can present information in an easy-to-understand manner			
Evaluating			
Checking the feasibility of ideas and ensuring all concerns and information are aired and debated			
Testing the consequences of a proposed solution (usually by discussion with the relevant people about what will be gained and what will be lost, searching for strengths and weaknesses of the proposal)			
Evaluating group performance (against task and relationship needs)			
Helping the group to evaluate its own performance against standards			

Features	Yes	No	Somewhat
External awareness			
I am aware of the history, recent changes and plans for the organisation			
I understand the current political environment in the organisation and the levels of government affecting my organisation			
I know the physical layout of the organisation and am aware of how that impacts day-to-day operations			
I know the current and forecasted economic environment for the organisation			
I know the social environment in which the organisation operates and the implications this has on how we deliver our service			
I know the values, strengths and personalities of the people that report to me and with whom I work regularly			
I know the values, strengths and personalities of the people I report to			

Functions	Yes	No	Somewhat
Internal awareness			
I am aware of my emotions and behaviour, particularly when I am in a stressful situation			
I know my values and needs			
I know my strengths and weaknesses			
The work that I do is in line with my values			
The work that I do allows me to utilise my strengths on a day-to-day basis			
I have a development plan to ensure I manage my areas of weakness and know to whom I can delegate these responsibilities			
Willingness			
I truly enjoy my leadership role			
I know how to use my personality and strengths for maximum, positive impact on others			
My self-confidence and self-esteem are both strong enough to enable me to handle criticism from others			
I am always on the lookout for ways to develop and improve the service we offer			
I am always on the lookout for ways to develop the people that provide our service			
I am focused on results and outcomes			

360° feedback

Remember that the purpose of doing this assessment is to raise an individual's awareness about their performance in a particular area of their work so that they may develop further, build on strengths or address a weakness.

Who should fill in the form?

Feedback from 360° means from all around you. This means colleagues, boss or bosses, direct reports, patients, other organisations (e.g. local primary care trust), allied clinical staff and administrative support staff. You should have at least two representatives from each group so that in total you have input from at least 10 people. The more participants that provide feedback, the more of an overall picture you will have. Bear in mind though that someone in-house has to collate this information or you must be able to pay someone external to do this. There's no point in getting people to participate and then ignoring the results. Abandoning the feedback process, or ignoring results, is a great way to irritate and create distrust among those who have been involved.

What should they be told?

Ensure that those participating in the feedback understand its purpose: it is to provide a foundation for a development plan. Because of this, it is vital that they provide objective and honest feedback. Engage a third party to organise the process including whether or not people wish to remain anonymous in order to gain the best quality feedback for you.

In order to receive such input it is often best to request that people put their name on the form. This will also assist with the 360° review when action plans have been implemented because you can compare baseline and review results from the same person.

If, however, people suggest they will only be honest if they remain anonymous then try to reassure them that their participation will not be known by the person receiving the feedback. The input from people genuinely concerned about reprisals is especially valuable, so ultimately if they will only anonymously provide the quality of feedback that you are seeking, then guarantee it.

What kind of feedback is valuable?

Ideally, you want both qualitative and quantitative feedback. A simple scale out of 10 will give you an easy measure, which can be reassessed. The qualitative information is vital in giving you suggested options that you can use in your action plan. Ask as many questions as you need but not so many that the people giving the feedback feel overwhelmed and compiling the answers becomes laborious.

Collecting the feedback

The feedback may be reported as a graph, a compilation of text or as numerical information. Bear in mind that you will be using this report to compare against a review in 6–12 months so graphs can be particularly helpful. If there are several people from the same group (e.g. admin support staff), averaging their grouped results is often the easiest way to present their information.

Receiving the feedback

Ideally, someone objective will go through the feedback with you in a completely confidential environment. That person could be an external coach, a GP appraiser or the practice manager. Whoever it is, they need to have the skills to help you handle any sensitive issues that may arise, to co-create your action plan and support you in implementing your plan.

As the recipient of the feedback, ensure that you review it with the attitude that all feedback is useful and not to be taken personally to make you miserable. It is all going to help you improve, which is why you sought feedback in the first place.

Creating your development plan

When you create your development plan, consider your strengths and weaknesses.

For those areas that you naturally struggle with (i.e. your weaknesses), aim for a level of 'competence' only.

For those areas that naturally come easily to you (i.e. your strengths), or areas that you are interested in, look for opportunities to develop them. The bulk of your action plan should *focus on* developing your *strengths*.

Monitoring progress and the 360° review

As with any plan, there should be goals and a time frame against which you review your progress to see if you are on track. Schedule time in your diary to review your progress over the period you have set to achieve your plan. These reviews may be more effective if done with the person who presented your feedback as they can help you deal with any obstacles that are coming up for you.

If you are not making the progress you had anticipated, then consider:

- Have you found it difficult to actually do what's on your action plan? If so, what has been stopping you?
- Are you being sidetracked by other more 'urgent' things, which make you forget your action plan?
- Do you have a limiting belief that is holding you back from doing what's on the action plan? Having extra support, a more regimented routine, a 'reminder to act' system or getting a coach to explore your limiting beliefs with you can all help in these situations.
- Have you set unrealistic goals? It may be time to readjust them considering the resources of time and energy that you have.
- Have people simply not noticed the changes you have made? Seek further input from other staff if you think your reviewers are inaccurate.

After six to 12 months of implementing your action plan, there should be a significant difference in the feedback you receive. Do your 360° review at the 12 months mark as a final evaluation of your progress. *See* Table 10.2.

Step 3: Goal setting

What to focus on

As mentioned, when you are creating your goals it is recommended that you focus on *developing* your strengths and *managing* your weaknesses. This is based on studies by Clifton and Buckingham, referenced in their book *Now, Discover Your Strengths*.[2] They demonstrated that business productivity and employee retention increased comparably with increases in the number of employees that could answer 'strongly agree' to the question: 'At work, do you have the opportunity to do what you do best every day?' They also found that 'the two assumptions that guide the world's best managers [are]:

1 Each person's talents are enduring and unique.
2 Each person's greatest room for growth is in the areas of his or her greatest strength.'

Consider for a moment how you feel about these assumptions. Do they make sense? What's the difference in how you feel when you think of doing activities that use your strengths compared with activities that you find difficult. For most people they look forward to and feel a lot more enthusiastic about using their strengths. It's quite simply more fun and more rewarding!

'Strengths' are defined by Clifton and Buckingham as those talents or things that we can consistently do to near perfection. You might be great at empathising with

Table 10.2 Sample 360° form using the 'traffic-light system' or 'start, stop, continue'.

360° feedback for Dr/Mr/Ms (insert name) _____

Date _____

Completed by (insert name) _____

Thank you for taking the time to give your honest feedback. Please be as specific as possible when writing your answers.

Q1 How would you rate XX at addressing inappropriate behaviour by staff members?

0	1	2	3	4	5	6	7	8	9	10

Very poor   Excellent

Please state one thing that you would like XX to *start* doing to improve how they address inappropriate behaviour by staff members.

Please state one thing that you would like XX to *stop* doing to improve how they address inappropriate behaviour by staff members.

Please state one thing that you would like XX to *continue* doing regarding how they address inappropriate behaviour by staff members.

Q2 How would you rate XX at building and maintaining positive staff relationships?

0	1	2	3	4	5	6	7	8	9	10

Very poor   Excellent

Please state one thing that you would like XX to *start* doing to improve how they build and maintain staff relationships.

Please state one thing that you would like XX to *stop* doing to improve how they build and maintain staff relationships.

Please state one thing that you would like XX to *continue* doing regarding how they build and maintain staff relationships.

Q3 How would you rate XX as a communicator of developments/changes affecting and occurring in the practice?

0	1	2	3	4	5	6	7	8	9	10

Very poor   Excellent

Please state one thing that you would like XX to *start* doing to improve their communication of developments/changes affecting and occurring in the practice.

Please state one thing that you would like XX to *stop* doing to improve their communication of developments/changes affecting and occurring in the practice.

Please state one thing that you would like XX to *continue* doing regarding their communication of developments/changes affecting and occurring in the practice.

Q4 How would you rate XX as a teacher of skills and processes for new staff?

0	1	2	3	4	5	6	7	8	9	10

Very poor   Excellent

Please state one thing that you would like XX to *start* doing to improve their teaching of skills and processes.

Please state one thing that you would like XX to *stop* doing to improve their teaching of skills and processes.

Please state one thing that you would like XX to *continue* doing regarding their teaching of skills and processes.

Q5 How would you rate XX for their awareness of what is happening in other teams in the practice?

0	1	2	3	4	5	6	7	8	9	10

Very poor   Excellent

Please state one thing that you would like XX to *start* doing to improve their awareness of what is happening in other teams in the practice.

Please state one thing that you would like XX to *stop* doing to improve their awareness of what is happening in other teams in the practice.

Please state one thing that you would like XX to *continue* doing regarding their awareness of what is happening in other teams in the practice.

Q6 Please briefly list other specific areas in which they could improve and which areas you think they are strong at.

Could improve in:

Already strong at:

people so they talk easily and openly with you, or creating strategies, or including people so they feel part of the group, or commanding so you are comfortable taking charge, or developing so you see the potential in people. When you are using these strengths you enjoy the task at hand and your performance is excellent most of the time. To formally identify your strengths take the StrengthsFinder profile in the book *Now, Discover Your Strengths*. For an informal evaluation you can do the exercise below.

Exercise: What are your strengths?

Answer the following questions on a separate page.

- What activities are you really good at? Consider your personal and professional life.
- What do you receive compliments about?
- What do you find really easy to do? Consider your personal and professional life: planning, looking at the big picture, creating the detail, bringing people together, making new friends, deepening existing relationships . . .
- What do you most enjoy doing? Coming up with ideas, starting projects, seeing things through to completion . . .

Look for the recurring patterns in your answers and list your top five strengths here:

Now consider how those strengths are used at work, how you could utilise them more or how you could introduce them.

How to set goals

There are certain features that, when embraced, make goals more likely to be achieved. They are 'POWER' goals:

- Positive/Present tense
- Own the goal
- What/When
- Effect/Evidence
- Resources.

Positive and present tense

Positive

This means you must state what you *do* want, not what you don't want. This is essential to your success as you get what you imagine. If you want to be less panicked, that means you still want to be somewhat panicked. Instead, what are the positive emotions you want to feel? How do you want to see yourself behaving? Your goal might instead be to feel relaxed and confident. If you have difficulty thinking of what you do want, write a list of what you don't want and then write the opposite next to each point.

Present tense

When we use words like 'wish', 'will', 'try' and 'hope' (e.g. 'I will try') we set up something for the distant future that may or may not happen. Instead, when we use the words 'am' and 'can' (e.g. 'I am a confident person') we tell our minds that this is happening now, which leaves no possibility for it to not happen.

Own the goal

Is this what *you* really want? Make sure your goal is something you 'want' to do, not something that you think you 'should' do (e.g. do you want to improve your presentation skills or do you think you should?).

'Want to' versus 'should do' goals

'Should do' is all about being pushed either by yourself or by someone else. This is really tiring and so hard to sustain that people usually give up. The alternative is to 'want to', which is about being drawn toward accomplishment.

For example, think of something that you really want to do. Picture that in your mind and take note of how you feel in that situation. Is your energy level low, medium or high?

Now think of something that you feel you should do. See it in your mind and notice how you feel. Note your energy level for this idea.

You will have felt a lower energy level or a weight on you in the second scenario, compared with the first. You can use this technique when evaluating your goals, by testing your energy levels. If they are high, go for it. If they are low, revise the goal.

Importantly, is the achievement of this goal within your control? If you have stated that you want your colleagues to carry more of the administration load, this is not within your control. If you wanted to be more effective at delegating or more efficient at getting your administration work done, then this is within your control.

What and when

What do you want to achieve and to what level?

When do you want to achieve it by? Putting a time frame around your goal will give you focus and clarity when you come to deciding the action steps to take.

Effect and evidence

Effect

What will be the effects of you achieving your goal on the important parts of your life (e.g. your relationships, career, happiness)? What else is important to you that may be affected?

Also, we often think in terms of what achieving goals will give us but there are usually things we will have to let go of as well. For example, if I wanted to achieve a certificate in teaching, I would also have to lose some of my recreational time. I have to ask, 'Do I really want to use that time for studying or for my hobbies?' If I'd rather be doing my hobbies, then I probably won't achieve that particular goal.

Ask yourself:

- If I do achieve goal X, what will I gain?
- If I don't achieve X, what will I gain?
- If I do achieve X, what will I lose?

Evidence

- How will you know you have achieved your goal or are on the right track?
- What will you see, hear and feel both external to you and in yourself?
- What are you achieving or doing differently?

From these features, you should be able to create a means of knowing if you have achieved your goal. For example, one of my clients used a traffic-light system to gauge his stress levels and noted that they had reduced from red to green in eight weeks. You could also aim for a certain increase in your 360° feedback scores or count how many days a week you get home on time.

Resources

What resources, internal and external, will you need to get your goal?

Your internal resources may include knowledge, skills and attitudes such as knowledge about how people process information, communication skills and an attitude of courage when you need to challenge difficult behaviour. Your external resources may include time, equipment and money.

Once you have identified the resources required, you can then decide which ones you already have, which ones you need to buy, which ones you might find in other people or which ones you need to develop for yourself.

What can goals be about?

Anything really, but broadly they usually fall into performance, learning and enjoyment.

You may want to focus on an outcome or performance:

- Receive positive feedback from 90% of my colleagues in the next 360° appraisal on how I handle conflict.
- Increase the amount of patient appointments per hour handled by the receptionists by 5%.

You may want to focus on learning:

- Notice the tone of the caller's voice to determine if they are in a positive or negative mood and mirror the energy and enthusiasm of the caller's voice when responding to them.
- Complete one module of a teaching course qualification in the next year.

You may want to focus on enjoyment:

- Feeling relaxed and confident 80% of the time when giving presentations.
- Enjoying interacting with patients.

Example of a specific outcome/performance goal

Goal

- To challenge negative behaviour by staff either on the spot or within one working day.
- Do this 95% of the time when this behaviour occurs.
- Achieve this rate in three months time. It's now January; I shall work on this until May when I will re-measure during that month.

Current situation

I challenge behaviour in this time frame only 30% of the time based on estimate/measurement over the past month.

Example of an enjoyment goal

Goal

Feel confident and relaxed when speaking during all staff meetings in three months time.

Current situation

Each time I speak during staff meetings, I feel panicked and anxious.

Turn to p. 96 for the Goals and Action Plan Form to record your work so far.

Step 4: Options for action

There are dozens of options to explore for achieving any goal. The best way to identify options is to look at the 'YOW' components which are **Y**ou, **O**ther people and the **W**orkplace. So, consider what can:

- 'you' do differently
- you do differently with 'other' people and what can 'other' people do differently to help you
- be changed in the 'workplace' environment (i.e. physical space, equipment and operating systems) to support you?

At this stage you need to create a long list of possible options. It is best to brainstorm in this section, which means don't edit your thoughts; just get them down on paper. Also, when you think you are out of ideas keep going until you have three more. Often these are the best ideas!

You

This means considering your strengths, beliefs, knowledge, skills and therefore what you can change in your thinking and behaviour.

Beliefs

Your beliefs influence your behaviour.

For example, if you believe that 'if you want a job done properly, you have to do it yourself' then you will be taking on all the projects and tasks that have to be 'done properly'. This will probably amount to most of your work, which will make you overwhelmed. In another context, if you think 'I can't be a good leader, because no-one listens to me' then you won't be confident when you speak to other people, so they won't listen to you.

A useful quote to remember by Henry Ford is: 'Whether you think you can or you think you can't you are right'.

Exercise: What are your beliefs?

To reveal your beliefs around leadership and other people, give at least three answers as you complete each of these statements.

I am a good leader because . . .

I can't be a good leader because . . .

As a leader I must . . .

As a leader I can't . . .

The people I work for are . . .

The people that work for me are . . .

To get the job done I . . .

Review your answers and ask yourself: 'Is this belief helping or hindering me?' 'Is it a true fact?' 'Does holding onto this serve my best interests?'

Highlight the beliefs that are hindering you and choose the three that are holding you back the most. Write them in the space below.

Old beliefs that hold me back

Do you need to modify these beliefs to help you achieve your goals?

Example 1

- 'To get the job done I must check what is happening every step of the way and keep control over the situation.'

As the leader you may still be responsible for the outcome but a more helpful belief would be:

- 'To get the job done, I must select the right person for the job, equip them with resources and confidence and be available only if they really need me.'

If you are a person who feels the need for control, these beliefs allow you to maintain a level of control that also gives others the opportunity to show their skills and build their confidence.

Example 2

- 'The people that work for me are incompetent.'

This belief is going to prevent you from delegating to and empowering your staff. You will be utterly overworked and your staff will be miserable.

This belief must be replaced by something more positive such as 'The people who work for me have untapped talents and capability'. If you believe this, you will believe that they always have something to offer you and can always improve as individuals and team members. . Test your new beliefs by asking again 'Does holding onto this serve my best interests?'

Write here your new beliefs replacing the top three that are hindering you and install reminders in your environment of your new ways of thinking. For example, you may want to imagine a member of staff holding a certificate (to show their capability) or you can use post-it notes with images or words.

New beliefs that support me

Knowledge and skills

The knowledge and skills that a person has changes frequently over time. Skills are developed through practical experience and usually involve learning a sequence of practical steps. For example, there are certain things to do in order to sensitively communicate bad news to patients or take a biopsy from a suspicious mole. These both involve the gaining of knowledge and development of skills.

Exercise: Building knowledge and skills

Thinking of your leadership and teambuilding role, what knowledge and practical skills would benefit you? Would better influencing or negotiation skills help you? Would it be helpful to have more knowledge of the current political climate? Would knowing more about your staff's strengths help you lead them? Would speed reading help you get through the paperwork you regularly have to read?

Remember you don't need to know or be able to do everything. Your team members are there to report relevant information to you and do particular tasks such that the whole team's cumulative skills and knowledge is adequate, if not in excess of the required levels.

What additional knowledge and skills do you want to develop to be a great leader?

Other people

Mixed messages

Sometimes we blame other people for the outcome of a situation when in fact the outcome is the result of our actions.

For example, the receptionist wasted your time when she wouldn't stop talking. But did you tell her that you had other things that you needed to do or was your body language saying 'I'm listening, keep talking'? The solution to this situation lies with you being assertive and not expecting others to miraculously know what you want them to do.

How does the other person want you to communicate with them?

Modelling your behaviour on the phrase 'Do unto others as you would have others do unto you' is a common, well-meaning mistake that we make when interacting with others. If you are a naturally quietly spoken, shy type of person, you've probably experienced interacting with a person who is louder and more intense. It's most likely that you didn't feel drawn to them and that you wanted them to be quieter and less 'over the top'. Alternatively if you are a louder person, you probably feel the urge to liven up quiet people and get them more involved. In fact, if we reflect back their communication style, we are likely to be more effective.

When we interact we tend to develop rapport more easily with people similar to ourselves. If you are a runner and you get chatting with another runner, there is usually an instant connection on a conscious level. You can also create rapport on an unconscious level based on body language, voice volume and energy levels. The point of developing rapport is that the connection it creates makes us more willing to listen to each other.

If you have difficulty communicating with certain people, try building rapport using these neuro-linguistic programming (NLP) techniques.

- Raise or lower your voice to be similar to their volume.
- Increase or reduce the energy in your voice.
- Match their body language. If they talk with their hands, then move your hands more in conversation. If they have their arms folded, cross your hands in front of you. If they are sitting relaxed back in their chair, do the same and don't sit on the edge of your seat leaning forward.

Similarly, how we convey information differs. Some people want the detail and background of a situation while others want to know bullet-point information and nothing more. When you aren't sure how much detail the person wants either ask them 'How much detail do you want me to give?' or pay closer attention to how they communicate with others.

Workplace

This means considering how your physical space, equipment and operating procedures can best support you.

Physical space and energy

I remember talking to a receptionist who had returned from a wonderful holiday. I asked her what she had enjoyed the most and she described the hotel. Its colour scheme and decorations had made her feel relaxed and calm while the open plan gave her the feeling of space to think.

This illustrates the power of colours, furnishings and layout of a practice upon the energy of the people in it. If you have your own office you have the freedom to decorate according to whether you want energising, relaxation or inspiration. Some people play music to relax after the morning surgery, others have photos of their family or reminders of holidays they have taken.

Physical space and information and relationships

The layout strongly affects the movement of information and relationships in an organisation. I know locum doctors who've reported feeling like 'outsiders', stating how they appreciated a communal area to meet other staff and to reduce their feeling of isolation. An area that can be closed off from patients, or other staff, creates privacy to facilitate private or confidential conversations.

The layout will also influence how easy it is to deliver messages and convey information. If there is a large physical space in which to work or the managers are all tucked away in offices, it is more difficult for them to be aware of the general goings-on in the day. This may however also be advantageous by making them less accessible for regular interruptions. A communal area for coffee and getting organised in the morning allows people to interact informally. What they talk about is not important; it's having that time and area to connect that is important.

You don't need to build extra rooms nor do major renovations; just think of what can be painted, added, moved, or taken away.

Another way to use your environment is to send relevant messages to colleagues or patients. A closed door, or a door with a 'do-not-disturb' sign on it, gives a clear message. If you are working in open plan, then try making a 'stop' or 'go' sign for your desk.

Some examples

A lot of general practices have space taken up with old patient files. It not only makes the practice feel cluttered but also makes this space unworkable for any other activities. While converting the paper to electronic files as a long-term solution, in the short term, storing files off-site can free up significant space.

Ask your patients what signs would give them better direction when moving around the practice or when waiting to see the clinician. I worked as a physiotherapist in a general practice and was located at the end of a long winding corridor. Part-way down, new patients wondered if they were still going in the right direction. A sign on the wall would have alleviated that confusion.

In an open-plan office area where I worked, the head receptionist was also out in the open and was consequently bombarded with interruptions. The bulk of these questions could have been answered by referencing a file or procedures manual but she knew it all so it was easier for us to just ask. Unfortunately, due to the limited space she couldn't be given her own office so the solution to this was for staff to recognise how disruptive these interruptions were and to reach for the manual or file instead.

Equipment and facilities

How often have you wanted to throw an inefficient, malfunctioning computer through the window? Investing in equipment that works effectively is crucial. It reduces stress for staff and gets the job done more quickly.

Good quality facilities also send a message to staff and patients. Clean waiting areas with comfortable chairs for those who've had hip replacements shows that you consider patient comfort to be important. In other words, you care.

For example: I was looking for a cup of coffee in a practice where I was facilitating a meeting, when a secretary came in to the kitchen. She helped me find what I needed to make a drink and noted that there was only instant coffee in this kitchen but the doctors had 'real' coffee. Her tone indicated her dissatisfaction with this arrangement. This simple difference was contributing to a sense of 'us and them' within the practice team. I wondered how much providing real coffee for the admin team would cost for a year compared with the cost of teambuilding workshops.

Operating procedures

These are the procedures that define how things are done in your department or business. They are meant to make life easier by creating a standard to work to but sometimes they become more complicated than necessary, are forgotten or don't even exist. For example, most businesses have procedures for inducting staff, registering new patients, inputting and collecting prescriptions, paying staff and taking disciplinary action. Often, though, there is a lack of procedures to deal with or prevent difficult interpersonal behaviour from staff or patients, taking excessive sick leave or for the doctors to do their clinical administration.

Your options for operating procedures are to introduce them, remind people of existing procedures or review and streamline them. Whenever you are creating or modifying, ensure that you receive input from all parties involved in the procedure. Not only are they likely to have the most valuable ideas and background information but it also creates greater commitment to the final procedure through ownership.

Step 5: Act and learn

Once you have created a long list of options, decide which ones to implement based on what will make the greatest positive difference, what the organisation is capable of doing immediately (i.e. all resources needed are already available) or what the people of the organisation are willing to do.

When you are deciding what options you wish to turn into action points, consider YOW and think in terms of what you or others can:

- stop doing and the new behaviour or thinking that will replace it
- start doing
- continue doing.

Opportunities for action

Once you have selected the actions you wish to take, consider when you will have the opportunity to actually do them. These opportunities will act as a trigger for you to practise your actions. For example, you may intend to start coaching others instead of solving their problems or doing the job yourself. The triggers to practise this action are when staff come to you with a problem, during staff meetings and when you feel the urge to solve their problems.

Rewards

At the end of the Action Plan Form in Table 10.3 you will notice a space for rewarding yourself. When people are making big changes, achieving results can often appear way into the future, making it hard to remain inspired. Think of the saying about how to eat an elephant. You take one bite at a time!

Give yourself rewards along the way as you do each little step. This will help you stay on track. Your rewards are completely up to you so have some fun with this as you brainstorm.

Writing goals will not change a thing unless you start to *do* something differently.

Table 10.3 Goals and Action Plan Form.

Date: _____

| Goal one | Target date |

Goal:

Current situation:

| *Action* | *Opportunities to practise* |
| What: | When: |

| Goal two | Target date |

Goal:

Current situation:

| *Action* | *Opportunities to practise* |
| What: | When: |

| Goal three | Target date |

Goal:

Current situation:

| *Action* | *Opportunities to practise* |
| What: | When: |

Rewards

This is the 'action' part of the process. You must be kind to yourself at this stage as regularly behaving or thinking differently to your 'normal' way takes time.

Learning

If you are overly critical of yourself you may be inclined to give up and revert to your old behaviours. Remember to reward yourself and maintain your learning approach. Do this by regularly asking yourself:

- Which of my actions have brought me closer to my goals? (These actions you will continue or do more frequently.)
- Which actions have not brought me closer to my goals?
- What have I learned from doing these actions?
- What other options do I have now?
- What changes, if any, will I make to my action plan?

The ISAGOAL process is a starting point and a means for continuing your development in any area.

When does the process stop?

When you want it to. Usually this means when you are happy with the skill or knowledge level you have developed or when the 'new' behaviours you have been practising become familiar ones. This whole process is really about taking a more conscious approach to learning.

Sounds like a lot of effort?

If all of this sounds like a lot of effort and you are not sure whether you will be able to sustain it, you are not alone. Having to keep yourself motivated during this period of learning and change is hard work but it can be made a whole lot easier by ensuring the other elements of your life actively support you. This needs a whole chapter to itself, which you will find in Chapter 14, 'Essential supports'.

Suggested learning outcomes and action points

1 Know what ISAGOAL stands for.
2 Know how to implement a 360° feedback process for personal development.
3 Practise setting POWER goals. Start with just one thing you would like to improve and be sure to ask other people for their suggestions in the options stage.
4 Add something to your environment that reminds you that 'all learning is valuable even when the outcome isn't what you hoped for'.

References

1 Robinson J. *Communication Miracles for Couples: Easy and Effective Tools to Create More Love and Less Conflict*. Berkeley, USA: Conari Press; 1997.

2 Buckingham M, Clifton D. *Now, Discover your Strengths*. London: Pocket Books; 2005.

Further reading

- Galwey WT. *The Inner Game of Work*. London: Texere; 2002.
- Becker F. *Workplace by Design: Mapping the High-Performance Workscape*. Jossey Bass Wiley; 1995.
- McGraw P. *Self Matters*. London: Pocket Books; 2004.

Chapter 11

Fundamentals of teams

What makes a team more than the sum of its parts?

Groups or teams

Today in our everyday working lives we often hear talk of 'workgroups', 'team members' or 'performing teams'. These terms are liberally sprinkled in conversations and everyone nods wisely in agreement or they just get on with solving the issues of the day, saying 'That's nice, but in the real world . . .'

It is important therefore to understand the differences between groups and teams and the significance teamwork can make to resolving a situation and/or achieving a desired outcome. If we did, we would probably choose our terms more carefully, particularly as we increasingly seek ways for making our working lives easier, more productive and more fulfilling.

There are clear distinctions between a 'group' of people and a 'team'. A group can be described as an aggregation of people with usually one simple thing in common (e.g. BMW drivers, lottery winners, employees of a general practice). There is usually no other connection between them.

A team on the other hand can be defined as a functioning unit of people who meet key criteria, namely:

1 members have work tasks that are **interdependent**
2 members are committed to **collaboration**
3 the team is **held accountable** and rewarded by the organisation **as a single unit**
4 the team will have a unique **charter** or an official mandate, something that **describes the reason for its existence.**

Not all teams are able to comply with all of these criteria, particularly in general practices. For example, health visitors and physiotherapists are usually employed by the primary care trust and are therefore accountable to their employers rather than the practices. However, for the practice to be successful, these professionals must collaborate closely as their work is interdependent with other roles in the practice. From these criteria, general practices include people with many disciplines. The key to it all is to fashion these members to work collaboratively.

In good teams, members have a sense of loyalty and belief in each other. Members need each other to help them do their respective work, to make work decisions, to solve problems, to make plans and to manage change. Also, imperative for teams to be effective is their successful balancing and integration of task behaviour (i.e. how people achieve the task) and relationship behaviour (i.e. how people are working together).

Team life-cycle

Unless you are setting up your own general practice or department from the ground up, you will have inherited a group or team. It is most likely that they have been 'thrown together' because of resources available at the time or a lack of knowledge about how to construct a team. As you read this section consider where your team or teams are in the life-cycle stages. Knowing this will help you begin to understand some of the dynamics and behaviours of your team(s).

Team life-cycle stages

In 1965, Bruce Tuckman[1] released the findings of his research into team formation and cycles. He devised an enduring model, as illustrated in Figure 11.1. It has since become a cornerstone of team development and understanding. Tuckman's model explains that as a team develops in maturity and ability, it will pass through and experience different stages of relationships, needs, leadership style and progress. As its purpose and/or composition changes over time, a team may well find itself recycling through various stages in this model.

Stage 1: Forming

As the title suggests, a team that has just been put together will commence in this 'forming' stage. It is safe to say that, from the start, the team behaves more like a group. Aggregated together under the title, for example, of 'Greenfield Surgery

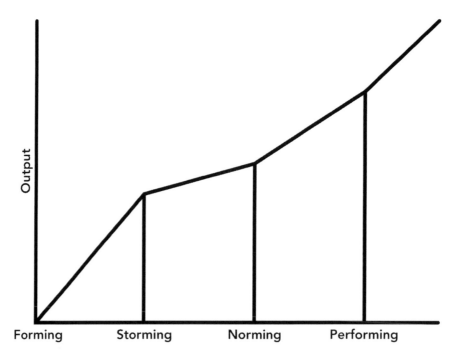

Figure 11.1 Stages in a team's life-cycle.

Nursing Team', the one simple thing they have in common at this early stage is that the nurses are employed by Greenfield Surgery.

This stage is characterised by a lot of testing activity. For example, members will test their understanding of each other and of the objectives for the team. They will ask lots of questions, particularly of the team leader. There is therefore high dependence on the leader for guidance and direction. Team goals and direction will come from the leader because individual roles and responsibilities are unclear. Members may also start to question why they are in the team, why they belong, what is expected of them as well as test the tolerance of the system and the leader.

If this testing activity reveals unsatisfactory or no answers, the team will not progress. However, as understanding grows, team members begin to settle and people find their relative place among the other members. Personal exchange and contact increases gradually with time and relationships start to build. An experienced team leader will also know that while this stage is quite amiable, caution remains a dominant feature for members and enthusiasm can often be tempered.

This forming stage naturally occurs and recurs when team members leave or new members arrive and when teams or groups of people are thrown together (e.g. two practices merging). It is important that this stage is given the attention it needs because it is fundamental to the team's future success.

There are no hard and fast timings associated with this stage and the leader has a significant role as controller and coordinator during this stage.

Stage 2: Storming

Synonymous with the title, this stage is characterised by infighting and friction. This may seem strange given the team has embraced positive behaviours towards the latter part of 'forming'; however, storming is beneficial. Disagreements will abound as members wrestle for clarity of purpose for themselves and for the team. Uncertainties can persist over task and task-related behaviours, over relative priorities of goals and also the role of the leader. Indeed the team leader may be challenged from team members as they vie for position and influence.

It is not uncommon for some members of the team to leave during this stage nor is it rare for the leader to lose effective control. Both of these outcomes can create an emotionally charged environment for the team in which to work and create an uncertain future.

The team therefore requires strong leadership, a commitment from its members to seek common ground and a focus on the team's goals and objectives to avoid being distracted by relationship and other non-objective issues.

If a group of people have come together (e.g. two practices merging) or a new member joins the partnership, the storming stage can either be the undoing or making of the team, dependent upon style of leadership and how quickly each member interacts and collaborates. Clearly, the team needs goals and objectives and corresponding roles and responsibilities for its members.

The leader focuses on coaching the membership, troubleshooting and providing a framework for the resolution of issues.

Stage 3: Norming

This stage characterises itself from its predecessors by the distinctly energising effect of getting everything and everyone organised. Team members begin to agree how the team will operate and about the information it requires in order to achieve its goals. The team leader will largely facilitate this behaviour and activity and strive for overall consensus among the membership. In return the team exhibits task-oriented behaviours and embraces compromise as it moves towards successful completion of its tasks.

While the task dominates the minds of its members, a norming team will also cement relationships where cooperation, empathy and positive expressions of support across the team occur. Roles and responsibilities have become clearer and are embodied by the membership creating a sense of commitment and unity. As the team defines and agrees its working processes and style, some aspects of the leadership become shared.

The leader spends time facilitating and energising the team, feeding back information in order to stimulate patterns of continuous improvement.

Stage 4: Performing

This may be the most enjoyable stage but it is certainly the hardest stage to maintain progress in. As the title suggests, the team has to focus on doing the work well. Founded on clearly understood roles and tasks and characterised by a sense of unity and closeness, the team nevertheless needs to continually ask and measure whether or not it is being effective and efficient. Becoming aware of the 'big picture' therefore is all important for the membership.

A willingness to understand the team's objectives and performance *within* the overall vision and goals of the organisation is a must for team members during this stage.

While the team now should have a shared vision and be able to make decisions independent of input from the leader, a set of criteria should guide effort, direction and results. The team owns its processes and systems and is able to develop and make changes where necessary; any disagreements are resolved positively and problems quickly solved. Along the way, relationships are strengthened and development needs of the membership addressed.

The leader focuses on delegation and generally oversees progress, occasionally advising team members when requested. Measurement of performance occurs and, as a unit, results and corresponding actions are agreed and implemented. Ideally decision making occurs by consensus; however, if this cannot be reached, the leader will have to make the final decision based on the information received from the members.

Revisiting stages of the life-cycle

A team may find itself revisiting any stage during its life-cycle if team composition changes or the task changes. For example, a team of doctors that includes trainees will be more susceptible to revisiting the forming and storming stages of the life-cycle as each new trainee arrives.

The same usually occurs if the task is changed; the team may return to storming or norming activity or even a combination of the two. For example, if the team that was created to implement the quality and outcomes framework (QOF) was then asked to create a new appointment system, their roles, purpose and responsibilities would need to be reviewed. People who perhaps had not participated as much in the first task may feel their opinion is more relevant to the second task and become more assertive and challenging. This change in behaviour is what stimulates the return to the other stages.

A team needs therefore to be flexible, adaptable and willing to embrace change as it makes use of its experience and lessons learned to achieve cohesion and fulfil its purpose. Such flexibility could be put to the test if members' fears of returning to storming are realised. Fears can be lessened by acknowledgement of this process, communication among team members about their concerns and taking action to resolve those concerns. The leader's role is to facilitate this process.

A team will progress through each stage on its way towards working effectively and efficiently. The length of time in which the team will remain in any one stage will be primarily dependent upon:

- style of leadership
- willingness and commitment of its membership
- the task itself, its priority and corresponding impact upon the overall success of the organisation as a whole
- the skills and experience of members of the team
- the manner in which a team is composed
- the personalities of the team members
- members leaving or new members joining.

What stage is your team at?

Observation of the team relationships and how well tasks are being achieved will reveal the stage that a team is at. Explaining the four stages to the team members will reassure them that uncomfortable behaviours are a necessary step to becoming a performing team. They can also decide which stage they are at and take ownership of making progress through the stages.

Team dynamics

The dynamics of any team are often the intangible forces that exist and operate between its members. They manifest themselves positively and/or negatively and can impact how well a team works together and ultimately if the task is completed successfully. These dynamics can be complex and can arise from a number of situations or conditions, particularly:

- environmental – layout of a room; availability and quality of support systems; stressors; organisational culture
- personal – previous familiarity between members; inclusion and exclusion; personalities
- leadership – style; communication; roles and responsibilities; support structures
- attitudinal – positive and/or negative behaviours; accountabilities.

Environmental dynamics

The presence of an open-plan style workplace can positively benefit the dynamics of a team because it facilitates open communication within the membership; each team member can observe when and how to support each other and the team can identify with its particular space. Contrast this with a workspace that may not support open-plan working, resulting in the membership being separated. Or the team members may be separated from their leader. The dynamics within the team will be different for each situation and might be hard to manage. Any weakness in the team could be minimised or amplified in any of these situations and will require vigilance across the membership. The leader should provide a forum to review the impact of the environment such as in a staff meeting. Suggesting 'what if' scenarios is a good way to explore options. (For example, what if we had a separate meeting area? What if we had partitions in the receptionists' work area?)

If the team is to work well together, support systems will need to be of a quality that enables effectiveness and efficiency. Reliable and easy-to-use technology is essential for ownership of tasks and roles. The dynamics of the team will be impacted by both the availability and quality of such systems.

There are many stressors in a workplace and the more that can be minimised or, better, removed, the more likely the team will align itself with its task.

For example: in many general practices the receptionists have a fairly open-plan workplace, where they greet and administer to patients as well as complete other administrative tasks. On the one hand, this environment is supportive. Consider a receptionist having to deal with a patient behaving aggressively. Someone is likely to observe this event and can offer support if needed. On the other hand, if a receptionist is doing administrative tasks at the front desk but not making appointments they are still likely to be approached by patients, which may then be interpreted as an interruption with the environment then becoming a source of stress.

Conversely, doctors in general practices usually have their own treatment rooms, but not necessarily an attractive meeting area to have lunch or chat with their colleagues. This environment for the doctors therefore can hinder the development of a strong team as they miss the opportunity to build relationships in a non-business context.

The physical environment also has a strong impact on attitudes and hence behaviours. When you walk into your office, do you feel yourself go into work mode? When you sit in your favourite lounge chair, do you feel more relaxed? When you enter a room that is clean, tidy and organised, how do you feel? A team will feel the same way about the layout of their environment and their position within it.

Personal dynamics

When members of a team, who are perhaps close friends, or have worked together for a long period, engage in close collaboration, others can have a sense of exclusion. While such behaviour is a natural consequence of friendships, if it is not communicated it can lead to divisive attitudes. This happens particularly if the needs of others are not recognised or where the collaboration excludes others.

For example: a nursing team that we worked with had a distinct division between the 'old' staff who had been at the practice for several years and the 'new' staff who had recently been employed and also happened to be more recent graduates. The division was largely created by the 'older' staff's attitude of not involving the newcomers in the running of the team. This apparently well-intentioned behaviour, to ease the load on them, unfortunately left the new staff feeling excluded.

The environment also plays an important role in inclusion and exclusion thinking. For example, physically separating team members from each other or inconsistently distributing technology can result in exclusion or a sense of unfairness. These feelings can then become the focus instead of the task.

Personality types will also affect how individuals relate to each other; whether they are introverts or extroverts, 'people-pleasers' or task focused. There are many different personality-type assessments (as discussed in Chapter 4). However, in a management team, Belbin typing is one of the most accepted, and is covered later in this chapter.

Leadership dynamics

The style of leadership is critical to the length of time it takes the team to progress through each of the various team stages (i.e. forming, storming, etc.). If the team leader leads by compulsion during the latter stages such as in performing, the team will not reach maturity. Likewise, if during storming, the leader fails to use compulsion and persuasion and adopts a detached attitude and abdicates responsibility, the team will endure struggles that are longer than necessary.

The more support a team is offered by its leadership, the better the dynamics will be. Similarly, the clearer the roles and responsibilities are for each team member, the quicker the team will achieve norming behaviour, support one another and assume some leadership duties themselves, particularly holding each other accountable for results.

As the leader, or one of the leaders, of a general practice, you will oversee multiple single discipline teams and draw them all together to function as 'the practice team'. Your main task is to stimulate and drive commitment to the purpose of the practice from which the appropriate behaviours and activities will follow. If you are a team leader, your role is to maximise the performance of your team and maintain their connection with the other teams and the practice as a whole. You are integral to the overall function of the practice team. Your other vital role is to ensure that overactive egos of individuals or teams do not inhibit the performance of other individuals or affect relationships between teams.

Further challenges arise when the single discipline teams within the practice are in different stages of the life-cycle. For example, the receptionists are 'performing' while the nurses are 'storming'. The best approach in this situation is to educate everyone about the team life-cycles so they have greater patience and understanding for the teams in their various stages. Also ensure the leadership styles are appropriate for helping the teams progress as quickly as possible.

Attitudinal dynamics

You could say that attitudes are a consequence of the previous examples. The better the leadership ability, the greater the inspiration and focus for the team members and hence the more positive will be the attitude of each team member. Similarly, the more effective the support systems and technology are, the less likely the team will be to adopt negative attitudes.

Having the right attitude to the team's task, strategy and relationships is critical to ensuring positive, honest and constructive dialogue among the membership. The most vital attitude is one of trust which means that people are willing to speak openly about their successes, mistakes, concerns and ideas without fear of personal criticism. They must be confident that any judgements will be directed at the information they present, not themselves.

Healthy dialogue involves fully listening to a person before seeking clarification, offering comments or questioning what has been said. Patrick Lencioni, author of *The Five Dysfunctions of a Team: A Leadership Fable*,[2] states that once trust is achieved, all information and thoughts can be shared and properly debated. The result is that team members then have a sense that they have been heard so their commitment to the final decision is very strong. With strong commitment comes greater accountability to the task and results then follow as a natural consequence. In short, positive attitude means positive behaviour means results.

Attitudes will therefore directly affect the level of individual and collective accountability that the membership will have to its tasks, failures and successes. The dynamics of a team can be managed constructively by recognising the natural way that people interact and determining what their motivations are. The team leader may have to intervene appropriately to ensure the dynamics return to or maintain a positive outlook and impact.

Management teams

This section looks at the importance of planning the composition of a team and in particular the link between behaviours, personality and roles within a team. This is valuable to consider when a partnership is recruiting a new member to the management team. It can also be used to assess whether the current match between personalities and roles is accurate or if it can be improved.

Personality and role combinations

Over a period of nine years, Dr Meredith Belbin and his team of researchers studied the behaviour of managers from all over the world to determine the effect of team-based business decisions on business outcomes. Specifically, the exercise was designed to identify how certain combinations of managers brought about certain effects, particularly financial outcome. The managers in the study were psychometrically tested, placed in teams of varying composition and then engaged in a complex management exercise. During the exercise, their different core personality traits, intellectual styles and behaviours were assessed and recorded. Over time different combinations of behaviour were identified as underlying the success of the teams, which were then named. The role of 'Specialist' has since been added.

These roles are:

- action-oriented roles – 'Shaper', 'Company Worker' (also known as Implementer), and 'Completer Finisher'

- people-oriented roles – 'Chairman' (also known as Co-ordinator), 'Team Worker' and 'Resource Investigator'
- cerebral roles – 'Plant', 'Monitor Evaluator' and 'Specialist'.

Overall, Dr Belbin discovered that in successful teams all roles were observed in action. He concluded that team selections required focus not only on technical skills and experience but importantly on correctly filling in the roles.

This work is relevant because it removes the pressure to find the ideal individual for a specific job. Instead, in Dr Belbin's mind, attention should be paid to the selection, development and training of teams. The following provides a snapshot understanding for leaders and managers when looking to improve an existing team or compose a new one. Detailed reading of Dr Belbin's book *Management Teams*[3] will reveal a treasure trove of further information.

As an introduction to his work, Tables 11.1 and 11.2 summarise the roles in terms of extrovert and introvert characteristics.

Dr Belbin concluded that people with particular personality characteristics are invariably attracted towards certain occupations. Additionally, the culture of organisations favours a particular type of person with managers often recruiting in their image as well as being under pressure to recruit a person who fits into the 'standard' mould. The problem that can arise with this approach is a lack of the personality types which Belbin deems necessary for a truly effective team. However, he suggests there is room for an organisation to employ all types of people,

Table 11.1 Extrovert roles. These are outward-looking people whose main orientation is to the world outside the group, and beyond the task(s) in hand.

Type	Typical features	Positive qualities	Allowable weaknesses
Plant (PL)	Individualistic, serious-minded, unorthodox	Genius, imagination, intellect, knowledge	Up in the clouds, inclined to disregard practical details or protocol
Resource Investigator (RI)	Enthusiastic, curious and communicative	Capacity to contact people and explore anything new. An ability to respond to challenge	Liable to lose interest once initial fascination has passed
Chairman (CH)	Calm, self-confident, controlled	Treats and welcomes all potential contributors on merit; strong sense of objectives	No more than ordinary in terms of intellect or creative ability
Shaper (SH)	Highly strung, outgoing and dynamic	Drive and readiness to challenge: inertia, ineffectiveness, complacency and self-deception	Prone to provocation, irritation and impatience

This table has been modified from 'Useful people to have in teams', p. 73 in Belbin 2004.[3]

Table 11.2 Introvert roles. These are inward-looking people principally concerned with relationships and tasks within the group.

Type	Typical features	Positive qualities	Allowable weaknesses
Monitor Evaluator (ME)	Sober, unemotional, prudent	Judgement, discretion, hard-headedness	Lacks inspiration or ability to motivate others
Team Worker (TW)	Socially orientated, rather mild, sensitive	Ability to respond to people and situations. Promotes team spirit	Indecisiveness at moments of crisis
Company Worker (CW)	Conservative, dutiful, predictable	Organising ability, practical common sense, hard-working and self-disciplined	Inflexible, unresponsiveness to unproven ideas
Completer Finisher (CF)	Painstaking, orderly, conscientious, anxious	Capacity for follow-through, perfectionism	Tendency to worry about small things; reluctance to let go
Specialist (SP)	Driven by the pursuit of knowledge and information; loves learning	Single-minded, self-starting, dedicated. Provides knowledge and skills in rare supply	Contributes only on a narrow front. Dwells on technicalities

This table has been modified from 'Useful people to have in teams', p. 73 in Belbin 2004.[3]

provided they are technically competent in the area for which they have been selected.

Some of Belbin's main conclusions are as follows.

- The attributes of a team always have to be assessed against the demands of the situation.
- The qualities of a person can override the type of behaviour implied by the title of the job.
- A Plant and Resource Investigator can occasionally be combined in one individual.
- As Plants gain experience, they are rarely moved because they become too valuable a resource.
- A successful Chairman thinks in positive terms and shows appreciation for those who accomplish their goals.
- A Chairman combines skilful use of resources with effective control.
- A Shaper will improve the performance of a complacent team but can be disruptive in a well-balanced team.
- A Shaper will seldom like working with another Shaper.
- A Company Worker identifies with the company and looks for goals in work that are aligned with the team.

- A Monitor Evaluator makes shrewd judgements but can have low drive because it is generally thought drive interferes with judgement.
- A Team Worker trusts and has strong interests in people, human interaction and communication.
- A Completer Finisher is prone to anxiety but has high self-discipline and finishes everything started.
- The most successful Completer Finishers have a strong secondary team role as Plants or Monitor Evaluators.

More generally, in looking at the value of team roles, Belbin found that although teams might succeed in capitalising on their collective strength, any shortcomings in performance usually reflect the fault inherent in their team composition.

Teams are a question of balance. What is needed is not well-balanced individuals but individuals who balance well with one another. Nevertheless, Belbin found that there must always be one person who is clever either analytically or creatively on any management team.

Ineffective management teams are classified by Belbin as falling into two types:

1 those which are products of culture (i.e. unacceptable performance epitomises faults to which the organisation has long been subject to) such as poor communication of strategy or vision.
2 those where no deeply rooted causes are evident but are linked to an unfortunate combination of circumstances (e.g. obstacles preventing individuals finding their preferred team role).

For example, someone in a team can potentially make a valuable contribution but may be prevented because his or her natural team role may not be required or because a stronger personality has taken it. You will probably have seen this occur during meetings that seem to be hijacked by one particular person or group of people. Either they know all of the answers or have a lot of criticisms to make, at which point other people at the meeting become quiet and don't participate. This is a disaster for a team that wants to be productive. Leadership is vital here to encourage everyone to share their thoughts. On a more one-to-one level, a manager may override a team member's concerns with a flippant 'You'll be OK'. It takes a strong character to respond with 'No, I won't, I need help . . .' and most people, in our experience, are more likely to simply be quiet and not mention it again.

More typically in teams, the unexpected failure can be attributed to poor allocation of resources (people, equipment, money) within the team. Teams who are aware of their collective and individual strengths and weaknesses find it easier to adjust to these factors.

Although the preferred role of a person never changes, the opportunity usually exists for people to perform more than one role. This is particularly helpful if the team is small. If you are creating a team it is therefore important to identify individual preferences for roles so that key roles can be filled first. Similarly for existing teams, a re-appraisal of who is filling what role can redress any imbalance between members. At this stage, there is merit in suggesting that people undertake a simple Belbin Self-Perception Inventory (SPI) to find out team role preferences among members. The SPI is available through the Belbin Associates website.[4]

In conclusion, Belbin found the main factors contributing to management team success are:

- the attributes of the person in the Chairman role
- the existence of a good Plant
- a range in mental abilities
- a spread in personal attributes laying the foundation for different team role capabilities
- finding and matching useful jobs and team roles that fit personal characteristics and abilities
- recognising and deciding to do something about a latent weakness and/or imbalance of talents.

Team size

The following conclusions about team size are particularly valuable if you are starting a practice partnership from scratch, or if the team size is changing due to retirement or recruitment.

- The number of members in a team will depend upon the quantity of work that needs to be done. (While this point may sound obvious, it doesn't imply that the more people you have, the more work you accomplish.)
- The larger the team, the greater are the unseen pressures that dictate conformity (i.e. time available for members to talk/contribute).
- The stronger the structure, the less tolerance exists in the team for deviating from agreed protocols, methods or policies.
- Ten or 11 members would appear to be large enough to provide variety but small enough for intimacy among members.
- Where decisions must be made, a team of six members proved effective (i.e. optimised levels of contribution, ensured shared ownership).
- A team of six offered a broad range of technical skills and team roles so that a high degree of balance could be achieved.
- A team of four can achieve a level of intimacy, involvement and excitement but may not necessarily correspondingly achieve full collaboration and the consequent results.
- A four-person team of whatever composition does not have the resources to handle all predicaments that occur. It is too small for a Chairman to be truly effective.
- Three people of high ability and complimentary skills could become very effective if they act in a unified way. But the three will become dependent upon any one personality/individual, the absence of which for any reason could halt progress.

Team size and environment

Dr Belbin found that certain physical factors and conditions can influence team size. He found that organisations often underestimate the need for suitable meeting rooms of an appropriate specification. For example, teams invariably expand to fill the rooms in which they are housed. This results in teams becoming ideal for the rooms they occupy rather than the purpose for which they exist. However, if teams have to shrink in order to fit into small rooms, an impression can be formed in members' minds that major decisions are made by small cliques.

Belbin recommends that for well-balanced teams, rooms and furniture that are ideal for the team's use must be made available. Holding a meeting in a room that doubles as a kitchen or at a table surrounded by food will not support the focus of the meeting. Similarly, when working on team development it is more effective seating people in a semicircle or at a round table than directly opposite each other across a desk.

In summary, when you are looking to maximise team performance consider:

1 the composition of the team in terms of personality type and individuals' preferred roles
2 the size of the team for the task, whether it's the partnership as it runs the general practice or a smaller team for a project
3 whether there are any obstacles to gaining high quality contributions from all team members such as poor leadership resulting in the team being hijacked by a dominant personality
4 completing a Belbin Self-Perception Inventory to identify individual's preferred roles and make adjustments accordingly.

Suggested learning outcomes and action points

1 Know the difference between groups of people and teams.
2 Understand the life-cycle of teams.
3 Evaluate which stage each team is in and offer the appropriate support.
4 Understand the impact of combinations of personalities and roles in teams.
5 Complete a Belbin Self-Perception Inventory.
6 Review the roles and responsibilities of team members and align them with preferences.
7 Seek staff input on the impact of working environments.

References

1 www.businessballs.com
2 Lencioni P. *The Five Dysfunctions of a Team: A Leadership Fable*. 1st ed. San Francisco, USA: Jossey-Bass; 2002.
3 Belbin RM. *Management Teams*. 2nd ed. Oxford: Elsevier; 2004.
4 Belbin Associates[R]: www.belbin.com/

Further reading

• Kayser TA. *Mining Group Gold: How to Cash in on the Collaborative Brain Power of a Group*. 2nd ed. USA: McGraw Hill; 1995.

Chapter 12

Assessing and maximising team performance

Getting the most from your team

Assessment of teams

At any stage of a team's activities, it is useful to be able to step back and evaluate how effective the team is at that moment. Is it functioning and, if so, how well? Or is it dysfunctional? In addition to the factors and conditions described earlier, there are many forms of evaluation, effected by two approaches:

1   self-assessment (i.e. how well is the team working; are relationships developing and tasks being completed)
2   customer assessment (i.e. how does the team come across to those who receive directly and/or indirectly from the team's activities).

An evaluation will consider the impact of direct outcomes from the team (e.g. what has the team physically produced/created) and from indirect outcomes (e.g. has the team introduced a new procedure that consequently saves time, improves patient relationships and/or enhances the surgery's reputation).

Self-assessment

There are many methods available for teams to carry out a self-assessment. Whatever method is chosen, the assessment should examine the characteristics of team effectiveness against an appealing standard, i.e. one that the team chooses to use to benchmark its own progress. An example of this qualitative analysis is illustrated in Table 12.1. It is possible to do a quantitative evaluation but it is far more complicated and the majority of practices will not do this, simply due to time constraints.

Once assessed, the team can collectively identify an action plan for development of any low-rated areas. For example, if tasks are being completed but relationships are poor or conflict is high, the assessment must lead to a deeper appraisal of the dynamics of the team. Highly rated items can be shared, celebrated and analysed in order to repeat elsewhere. Knowing how a good result from a particular task has been achieved can lead to repetition on other tasks.

Customer assessment

Customers can be defined as all those people who directly receive something from the team's activities, whether it is documents, reports, treatment or something less

Table 12.1 Team self-assessment.

		All of the time	Some of the time	Hardly ever
Task and goals	Well understood, agreed and accepted. Clear assignments are made and owned by team members.			
Commitment and accountability	All tasks and agreements are taken seriously. Team members hold each other accountable for actions and results and question each other on inappropriate behaviour or inattention. Each team member is conscious of the team's function and objectives and periodically measures its own performance.			
Communication	Participation in discussion and action is high. Depth of communication is good, including ideas and feelings. No-one feels like they are holding back. Everyone feels that their thoughts are fully listened to.			
Conflict	Critiques are focused on ideas, processes and methods. Judgements are not made on personalities and people. Conflict is encouraged so that all thoughts are aired.			
Organisation	Meetings are well prepared, run and recorded. Decisions are owned, documented and promptly issued. Minutes are issued within an agreed period of the meeting.			
Decision making	Outcomes are viewed as beneficial and contributory to the organisation. Decisions are well informed. Aim for consensus decisions, otherwise agree the team leader will make the decision.			
Vision	Inspiring and energising. Agreed, documented and communicated. Communicated and referred to whenever relevant (e.g. decision making, during meetings)			
Environment	Supportive and complimentary. No-blame attitude. Business processes enable activity such as effective IT, efficient administration, well-organised team meetings. Risk taking is encouraged and mistakes are seen as learning opportunities.			

tangible such as encouragement and support. The customers of the management team are therefore the other practice staff members, the patients and other organisations such as the primary care trust.

Analysing the quality of the work being produced by the team can be a difficult activity, particularly when recipients of such work are a mix of people internal and external to the organisation. However, this can be a very accurate way to highlight successes and areas for improvement and is therefore worth the effort.

Someone on the inside who knows the objective of an idea, and the trade-offs that may have had to be agreed to get the idea off the ground, might view its success differently from someone with an external frame of reference. For example, if staff and management have had to make sacrifices in order for the new idea to become reality, they may hold some resentment to the outcome, or alternatively be even more proud of the results. Patients receiving a better service as the final result, however, would have only positive feedback. Consequently, assessment from internal and external sources is more accurate and comprehensive.

Generally, the main measures of quality are timeliness (e.g. is the report written or the new process in place on time), cost (e.g. did the new idea cost the surgery more than was budgeted) and functionality (e.g. does the new procedure do what it is supposed to do).

An assessment of the quality of work from the viewpoint of someone internal to the organisation needs to involve all of the factors accompanying the decision that led to commencement of that work. For example, if the quality of a new IT (information technology) system is being measured, its functionality (ability to fulfil its function), benefit (to users), cost (to the organisation) and timeliness (how long until it was ready to use) need to be considered.

For those customers who are external to the organisation (e.g. patients), measurement of benefits received from the team will use different parameters even though they can still be categorised in terms of timeliness, cost and function.

Consider the example of introducing a patient service that allows them to email repeat prescription requests. The surgery may be interested in measuring the quality of the process internally in terms of whether it allows patients to acquire their correct medication (functionality) and whether it affects the amount of time the staff take to dispense medication (i.e. cost of labour). External assessment by the patients however would focus on their satisfaction with the ease of ordering their medication.

Maximising team performance

For many organisations, having teams perform to their best can mean the difference between success and failure. Some general practices manage to survive but at a cost to personal relationships and professional development. Teamwork is the cornerstone of successful operations in any walk of life and so maximising team performance, within the context of a practice's overall vision and objectives, is crucial to everyone.

Essentially, maximising team performance requires:

- appropriate and good leadership, particularly from team leaders and management

- team members who know and accept what they are required to do
- team members accepting the standard to which they behave and work
- team members being responsible for what they are supposed to do
- team members being accountable to each other
- team members collaborating and helping each other
- an appropriate balance between focusing on the task and on building relationships.

Essential elements for a performing team

There are a number of essential elements that need to be established and agreed for a team to start working effectively. When properly implemented, they provide a firm footing for the team to perform and to improve on a continuous basis. These are:

1 vision
2 roles
3 responsibilities
4 leadership
5 deliverables and outputs
6 reward and recognition procedure (for individuals and the whole team)
7 team charter.

Vision

Many different terms are used by people to define what they believe is a 'vision', such as mission statement, strategies or goals. James Collins and Jerry Porras highlighted in their article 'Building your company's vision'[1] that there is a relevant difference between all these similar-sounding terms and that of 'vision'. Many enduringly successful organisations have a set of core values and a core purpose that never change even as their business strategies and the way they work may change to meet new demands and/or new regulations. It is the ability of an organisation to know what to preserve and what to change in order to remain effective that allows it to establish and honour a true vision. The vision therefore provides guidance on what focus to preserve and on the future in order to energise progress toward it. It provides the context in which the organisation operates.

The well-thought-out vision comprises two fundamental components, namely core ideology and envisioned future.

- Core ideology simply defines the enduring character of the organisation; it is what the organisation stands for and why it exists. This is a consistent identity that remains the same even in the face of changing demands, regulations, leadership or staff. It provides the glue for an organisation over its lifetime. It is itself made up of two elements:
  - core values are the essential and enduring beliefs of the organisation
  - core purpose represents the reason for the organisation's existence. It is not a goal or business strategy because either will change over the lifetime of an organisation; the core purpose remains unchanged.

- Envisioned future is what the organisation aspires to become, achieve or create. This aspiration will always require progress and effort to attain. It comprises a challenging goal and a vivid description to make it come alive:
  - challenging goals are needed to progress the organisation towards its future
  - a vivid description is needed to inspire and allow people to imagine what it will be like to achieve the goal.

A great example of a challenging goal was delivered eloquently by President JF Kennedy in 1963 when he announced his country's goal of putting a man on the moon and safely returning him to earth by the end of the decade. This clearly was achieved and the organisation responsible was NASA. Their updated vision 'Into the Cosmos' states: 'The vision for Space Exploration calls for humans to return to the moon by the end of the next decade paving the way for eventual journeys to Mars and beyond.'

Core ideology is reflected in space exploration requiring innovative science, at the heart of NASA. Envisioned future is covered by 'Mars and beyond'. Simple, but everyone knows what's ahead.

The Institute for Health Improvement(IHI)[2] defines its vision more specifically.

The IHI is a 'non-for-profit organization leading the improvement of health care throughout the world'.

> IHI is a reliable source of energy, knowledge, and support for a never-ending campaign to improve health care worldwide. The Institute helps accelerate change in health care by cultivating promising concepts for improving patient care and turning those ideas into action.
>
> We will improve the lives of patients, the health of communities, and the joy of the health care workforce. We will accelerate the measurable and continual progress of health care systems throughout the world toward:
>
> - safety
> - effectiveness
> - patient-centredness
> - timeliness
> - efficiency
> - equity.
>
> We will be a recognized and generous leader, a trustworthy partner, and the first place to turn for expertise, help, and encouragement for anyone, anywhere who wants to change health care profoundly for the better.

Roles

As is the case with players on a strong rugby team or employees in a well-run company, team members fill specific, defined roles. Building on Belbin's work, these roles need to be defined and agreed in the case of new teams and validated/reviewed for existing teams. Usually in filling these roles, some might volunteer for positions, some might be elected by the group, and others appointed by a manager. Some teams witness members assuming roles, without any due process at all.

Nevertheless, for all teams:

- there are a number of fundamental roles required for the team to perform effectively
- roles should be specific and defined but interdependent
- there are informal as well as formal roles to be filled
- not all roles need be filled all of the time.

Responsibilities

As distinct from roles, responsibilities are commitments made by team members to the successful completion of a task. These responsibilities arise from the accurate allocation of skills, strengths and experience. Once a role has been filled, responsibilities for the completion of particular activities and outputs should be agreed and documented.

For example, team leaders are responsible for moving the team to accomplish its task(s) by focusing members on the purpose and the end result required within the overall vision and agreed plans. Team leaders should facilitate an environment that supports and helps teams get their work done. One of the most important responsibilities of the team leader is to recognise and celebrate accomplishments and to communicate progress to the rest of the organisation.

To identify the roles and responsibilities, a good sequence of questions to ask is: 'What is your purpose within the practice?', 'What tasks must you do to achieve that purpose?' and 'What must you do to achieve that task?'

For example, a practice nurse would probably answer those questions with the following:

> My purpose is to provide excellent nursing care to the practice's patient population.
>
> The tasks I must do are: run the triage clinic, arrange the flu vaccinations, assist the doctor with the baby clinic, coordinate and deliver general nursing care . . .
>
> To achieve those tasks: I must effectively liaise with the receptionists, dispensers, secretaries, doctors and the practice manager, maintain up-to-date training, be active in looking for ways to develop our service . . .

Leadership

A good team leader uses combinations of the leadership styles to support and guide the team through its four stages. As noted, it is necessary for teams to move through each life-cycle stage in order to reach the performing stage; the leader has enormous impact on whether or not this is achieved.

During forming, the team members need to understand their purpose, roles and goals. This need is best met with leading by compulsion where this information is spelt out. During storming and norming, the leader's role is to support and encourage constructive conflict as roles, values, strategies and actions are developed and come alive. A mix of the styles is therefore needed; compulsion to remind members of agreed standards, support during disagreements, example to model expected behaviours and coaching to elicit participation and creativity. During the performing stage, the style is predominantly leading by example, trust, and coaching and support. These styles will also be strongly demonstrated by the membership to each other in this stage.

Deliverables and outputs

Whatever task has been set, the team will deliver something – a service, a document, some tangible output – to someone. This output will be measured by its recipient(s) and its standard evaluated in a conscious or sub-conscious manner. It is good practice for teams to agree at the outset what will be delivered by the team to whom and to what standard. In this way, the team can start to measure its output, monitor satisfaction levels from those on the receiving end and therefore engage in a continuous improvement regime. This does not mean having to micro-manage the team's outputs to the nth degree; rather it means the team having a good idea of its progress through self-monitoring key items. The lack of standards creates confusion and room for argument about whether or not a task is completed. If a standard is not set, everyone will establish their own individual standards, which often is not to the overall required level.

Reward and recognition procedure

One of the essential functions of leadership is to be able to recognise and reward achievement. Within the team environment, members will be focusing on achieving their individual tasks as well as ensuring the overall team goals are met. Team members should also be aware of each member's contribution to the team's success and have a procedure for recognising and rewarding such contribution. The levels of reward, to be determined by the team, can range from regular verbal/written appreciative recognition to a tangible monetary or gift reward.

The crucial aspect is for the team to identify and agree how decisions concerning recognition and reward will be made. They must then be consistently implemented for the system to be credible and to incentivise performance. Clearly any recognition and reward procedure must match the practice's resources, culture and circumstances and be relevant to the team's goals and objectives.

You should be wary of unfairly rewarding individuals who are not performing. Rewarding low performance removes the drive for people to work to a higher standard. This aspect of leadership does not entail becoming personal. It means that reward and recognition should fit the bill and so if an individual has not performed as anticipated, the team leader needs to ascertain the reasons. These may be situational (e.g. resources not available for the particular period needed or perhaps the individual has experienced a bereavement) or they may be innate (i.e. the task is new to the individual who has low confidence to achieve it). Having found out why, the team leader can work with team members and the individual to find a win-win solution.

Team charter

Having a team charter is a very useful way of cementing and then documenting the elements discussed above. The charter signifies each team member's pledge or agreement made to each other for the duration of the team's activity. It is particularly useful for new team members, for reminding team members of their commitments and also when communicating to others the reason for being on the team. It should comprise these essential elements:

- vision (including values and purpose, goals and vivid descriptions)
- roles
- responsibilities
- deliverables and outputs
- reward and recognition procedure.

The charter focuses on the end results and the standards to be maintained while getting there. If someone asks you 'How do you all work so well together?' your response should be 'This is how' and present the charter. This can be in the form of words or illustrations on a flipchart, a Mind Map[R]3 style diagram or a typed document. The point is that it should be documented so that everyone has this point of reference.

Table 12.2 Impact of obstacles on task and relationships.

Missing element	Impact on task achievement	Impact on team relationships
Vision	Lack of direction for the team; difficulty keeping on track; reduced likelihood of task achievement.	Arguments over goals; uniting against the management team who created the working team.
Roles	Lack of purpose for team members; difficulty focusing on work at hand; likelihood of finding other inappropriate or conflicting activities.	Poor commitment to collaboration; likelihood of interference and increased feeling of distrust.
Responsibilities	Lack of optimum utilisation of resources and people; skills and strengths unused; members drift.	Likelihood of members losing key skills and developing/ focusing on weaknesses; dependence upon team leader resurfaces.
Deliverables and outputs	No measures by which performance can be determined; lack of correlation between task setting and achievement.	Likelihood of low confidence and levels of morale; reward and recognition becomes unfocused and diluted.
Reward and recognition	Initial gains on task completion start to fall off; likelihood of incomplete tasks and/or task completion to lower than agreed standard.	Likelihood of members becoming unmotivated; indiscriminate and unfocused recognition leads to distrust and dissatisfaction; likelihood of staff turnover increasing.

Obstacles to team performance

It is worth indicating at this point the likely impact on task achievements and relationships that may arise when some of the key elements for team performance are absent. Table 12.2 illustrates some of these impacts.

Balancing task achievement and relationships

As described earlier, leadership can be embraced at any level of an organisation and be independent of role; any member of a team can assume leadership to ensure the effectiveness of the team. This is particularly important in the early stage of a team's development.

Chapter 11 introduced the staged life-cycle that a team is likely to progress through. How easily depends upon a number of factors. Therefore, one of the prerequisites for working as a team is to go through the process of becoming a team. Expressed previously in terms of 'forming', 'storming', 'norming' and 'performing', team development must incorporate people and tasks and interpret the relationship between them both. John Jones and William Bearley established the importance of this two-dimensional nature of team development in 'Facilitating team development: a view from the field'.[4]

Jones and Bearley identified the two dimensions as:

- Task Behaviour (i.e. how the team achieves the task)
- Relationship Behaviour (i.e. how the team works together).

Their work provides teams with a means for diagnosing where they are in relation to these two dimensions so as to get back or stay on track to developing the conditions in which effective teamwork thrives. For example, a team may choose to focus on getting the job done at the expense of team relationships or it may prefer internal calm for a while by sacrificing the task.

Different needs will feed different emphasis on task or relationship. Reasonable justification can be found for any emphasis. The important thing for a team and a team leader in particular is being able to recognise where it is in terms of task–relationship and why a particular emphasis is preferred over another. In many ways, considering these two dimensions advances understanding of the life-cycle of teams a little further because it observes task–relationship behaviour.

As Jones and Bearley conclude, when looking at task behaviours, at the outset of a team, members will start to identify what is required of them, identify resources and understand expectations placed on them. Once the team collectively understands its task requirements, it organises itself to achieve clearly defined goals. Having established a plan on how to achieve its goals, the team shares information, opinions, feelings and establishes good networks and communication channels. The advanced phase means the team is collectively managing the implementation of the decisions made.

We highlighted in Chapter 11 the impact that personality has on a team. While it may seem important to focus on Task Behaviours, the personalities and personal agendas within a team, especially in the early stages, may combine to undermine the achievement of a task. Therefore, understanding Relationship Behaviour is as important.

Accordingly in the life-cycle of a team, members are initially dependent on the team leader to explain task requirements and to energise common commitment to shared goals. Later, conflict arises where members vie for leadership and influence. This phase has to be faced by the team if it is to progress. Having resolved any areas of conflict, the team will experience relief and satisfaction, becoming more cohesive and increasing mutual respect and shared accountability. Eventually the levels of trust are sufficiently high that the team is confident to reorganise itself according to ongoing needs and to operate even in the absence of leading members.

An example of where emphasis would be placed on task achievement is the case of a practice moving location. During the actual move to the new building, every member of the practice will have specific tasks to complete in order for the move to be completed smoothly, effectively and within the required timescale. There will not be much time available to focus on relationships; suffice to say that everyone will need to collaborate. Conversely, consider developing a triage clinic where the nurses start performing some tasks previously done by the doctors. There will be a strong need during the development stage for support, coaching, training and trust so the relationships take priority. Without strong relationships, if the nurses struggle with the task they may be uncertain about seeking help and support, which could affect patient care, their own stress levels and the other teams involved in the clinic.

Collaboration

Collaboration will not guarantee your team success; however, not having it will severely impair a team from reaching its goals and from enjoying itself in the process. Thomas Kayser's book entitled *Building Team Power*[5] focuses entirely on the benefits and power of collaboration. Admittedly the book is aimed at the non-medical world; nevertheless the concepts and practical examples it contains are applicable to any body of people engaged in teamwork.

In his book, Kayser lists a number of themes of collaboration assembled from interviewing several managers and leaders in industry. This list presents examples of what collaboration looks like and feels like in a variety of forms. In his list, collaboration means:

- creating unity in the production of ideas, decisions, strategies, services, products, etc., so that the group is greater than any individual could achieve working alone
- having shared goals or priorities and working together to achieve them
- sharing and processing information – free from hidden agendas – in the pursuit of consensus
- setting aside one's ego to expand the human potential of others
- relying on each other for advice and counsel.

One interviewed person defined his measure of collaboration as a ratio of 'we's' to 'I's' that he hears in his interactions with people throughout his company. So if you are hearing more 'we's' than 'I's', there is a good chance that collaboration is alive and well in your organisation.

Collaboration has been a mainstay in Japanese culture for many years. The Japanese have the term 'Kaisen' at the root of their quality movement and it means gradual, unending improvement, doing little things better, setting and achieving higher standards. In this spirit, all organisations have a challenge to identify what they need to do to raise their level of excellence.

Collaborative working would suggest that a more facilitative approach to leading or managing a team is required. More and more people are becoming technically more expert than perhaps their managers. These people are also closest to the customer, end-user or recipient of the service provided. This makes team members the ones with wisdom and ideas about how to improve things. A primary role for managers and team leaders therefore will be to facilitate the use of this wisdom collaboratively by:

- asking the right questions
- encouraging team members to find the answers, especially within themselves
- encouraging sharing of information among team members
- increasing delegation
- increasing shared decision making
- encouraging empowered behaviours
- encouraging collaboration across cross-functional teams.

Like all appraisals, assessing your team's performance should bring few surprises if you are in tune with both the task and relationships. A well-defined, agreed and communicated charter enables collaborative working, which in turn takes the angst out of working.

Suggested learning outcomes and action points

1 Ask each team to conduct a self-assessment.
2 Compare self-assessment results against customer assessment (patient satisfaction surveys or feedback from other practice teams).
3 Create a team charter for the whole practice.
4 Revise your existing team charter or practice vision and make it more meaningful.
5 Communicate your charter or vision more often.
6 Get to know the emphasis placed on tasks and relationships and check it is right for the moment. Be flexible and focus on each one when it is needed.
7 Identify the extent of collaborative behaviour and listen out for the 'we's' against the 'I's'.

References

1 Collins JC, Porras JI. Building your company's vision. *Harvard Business Review.* 1996; Sept–Oct: 65–77.
2 www.ihi.org/ihi/about
3 www.buzanworld.com
4 Jones EJ, Bearley WL. Facilitating team development: a view from the field. *Group Facilitation: A Research and Applications Journal.* 2001. 3: 56–64.
5 Kayser TA. *Building Team Power: How to Unleash the Collaborative Genius of Work Teams.* USA: McGraw-Hill; 1994.

Chapter 13

Fixing dysfunctional teams

You've built and led a team. What happens if it's broken?

How to fix dysfunctional teams

Dysfunctional teams exist in general practice in two forms. There are either individual teams that are not functioning or there is an 'us and them' feeling between teams. We believe that the fundamental reason for such dysfunction is a lack of performance in the leadership functions (highlighted in Chapter 3), brought on by a leader with insufficient confidence, knowledge or skills.

When individual teams are dysfunctional it is often because:

- individuals have been allowed to behave inappropriately
- there is an absence of appropriate standards for behaviour
- there is no vision or purpose for that particular team
- roles are poorly defined and therefore argued over
- there are no performance goals
- individuals' needs are not being met
- reward and recognition processes are not in place or are unfairly applied.

When there is a feeling of 'us and them' between teams in the practice, it is often because:

- the needs of the team(s) are not being met (e.g. recognition of the receptionists' role in managing difficult patients or valuing the input from the nursing team in how to run clinics)
- of poor relationships, which are usually due to a lack of trust. A team that has been led by compulsion for too long doesn't trust their leader to grant them a degree of autonomy. A team may also have experienced leaders who don't practise what they preach or demonstrate double standards, creating a well-founded lack of trust
- the team has lost/been allowed to lose its focus on the vision of the practice and their role in supporting and realising that vision
- a personality in the partnership or management team has become the focus of the practice rather than the vision and purpose. This allows room for personality clashes where a team may act with an attitude of 'We don't like you, so we won't do XYZ'
- the ego of the team has been allowed to take priority over the needs of the task. It is vital that the leader regularly reminds the teams of their interdependence and that no one team is more valuable or favoured than another
- the team leaders are not fully committed to the decisions by the partnership/ owner and convey their dissatisfaction to the team members when they pass on

the information. This is a form of sabotage and team members are likely to lack commitment

- a cohesive front is not provided by all members of the management team including team leaders. Any disagreements must occur in private otherwise the strength of the management team is questioned allowing for favouritism and inconsistent standards of behaviour.

Step 1: Get to the root of the problem and identify what needs are not being met

Techniques for exploring a problem have already been covered in detail and can all be used in this situation. If there are very poor relationships between the teams and they are unlikely to be open and honest with a facilitator from within the practice then you will need an external facilitator or mediator. Ideally, meet with each team individually before bringing them together. This serves the purpose of allowing the teams to feel heard and understood by the mediator, gives an example of the process that will be used when the teams meet and reveals the needs of the teams to the mediator.

This also applies to dysfunction within a single team. A member of the practice is more likely to be able to mediate between factions or individuals in a team but they must be able to remain neutral and be independent.

Once the needs that are not being met are identified, they must be acknowledged by the other team or individual. This can be encouraged by saying 'Tell me what needs they said are not being met'. It's amazing how people hear completely different things to what is actually said. For example, 'I don't feel that my work is acknowledged' is heard as 'She says I never say anything nice to her'. Persevere until each party has demonstrated that they've heard correctly what the other has said.

Step 2: Create a strategy to meet each party's needs

Once Step 1 has been achieved there are usually two outcomes.

First, the needs identified can be directly addressed and the problem will be resolved. For example, if someone says they have the need to be recognised, ask 'What needs to happen in practical terms for you to be recognised?' Once some options are suggested, seek agreement between the two parties as to which ones they will implement.

Alternatively, the needs that have come up may not appear to be directly related to the problem. For example, you may be mediating between the nurses and doctors teams regarding problems in the running of a triage clinic, which the nurses are primarily responsible for. The nurses may seem to go off on a sidetrack stating they want recognition for the hard work they are doing throughout the practice. Once the doctor's team acknowledges this, the nurses may be more likely to discuss the existing problems.

When developing the elements of the strategy use the YOW tool to identify what skills and knowledge may be needed for all of the other people involved and what changes can be made in the workplace.

Step 3: Monitor adherence to the strategy

Strong leadership is needed here to prevent a return to the old behaviours that created the problems. Encourage all the individuals involved to hold each other accountable to the agreements made, while acknowledging that changing behaviour can be difficult. As part of the strategy, set dates and times for reviewing progress and do not let them be ignored.

Step 4: Simultaneously develop team relationships

It is always valuable to invest in developing stronger relationships between team members and if you have a dysfunctional team it is even more important. There is no point pursuing results or increased commitment from a group of people that do not trust and respect each other. They need to be able to share information about themselves, their successes, concerns, bright ideas and mistakes and will only be able to do that in an atmosphere where they trust they will be listened to and acknowledged and not be personally attacked.

Teambuilding can be done informally during lunch breaks and meetings and formally during time expressly protected for that purpose. Teambuilding games can be fun but are pointless if there is no reflection on lessons learned from the experience or follow-up. Patrick Lencioni's book *The Five Dysfunctions of a Team: A Leadership Fable*[1] has a workbook[2] companion which provides excellent exercises on building trust, mastering conflict, achieving commitment, embracing accountability and focusing on results.

For example, the 'personal histories' exercise for building trust asks team members to explain where they grew up, how many kids were in their family and what was the most difficult or important challenge of their childhood. These seemingly simple questions open up a dialogue on a different level to the chit-chat that usually occurs while making coffee at work.

Completing personality assessments as a team also gives valuable insights into why people behave the way they do. Having individuals share how they deal with conflict and difficult communication scenarios as well as exploring the reasons for their style allows for greater understanding between team members. This understanding is one of the biggest supports for team building. Too often people will think 'They are just being difficult', 'They're trying to make my life or this situation harder' or 'Why don't they just get what I'm trying to say?!'

A very simple tool for increasing commitment to an idea or action is to always clarify what people think they have just agreed to. Five minutes before the end of a meeting, check in with people to see what they think has been decided. Clarify any misunderstandings and then end the meeting.

We recommend Lencioni's book, over those that consist of teambuilding games, because it is more practical for general practice.

What to do if a dysfunctional team refuses to change

In these situations, team members' refusal to change usually surrounds negative behaviours they are unwilling to give up. As stated before when handling difficult behaviour by staff, termination of their position is sometimes the only resolution. In the following example from a corporate environment, people were moved to other departments, but this is often impossible in small practices.

For example: a multidisciplinary team was tasked with managing technical and building services (e.g. maintenance, project management, cleaning, reception, telephones) to a client's portfolio of office buildings. A lot of the work involved fixing problems as well as working to prevent faults and equipment breakdown. The leader inherited a team of skilful people who were not performing to the standards required of them.

The reasons were many, including:

- no vision available
- no clear roles and responsibilities
- no goals set
- distrust between team members and a demanding client
- no agreed standards of behaviour.

A lot of these situational issues were solved over time. However, the team had become so entrenched that a small subset of the team had formed into a clique. This small group could be observed to be extremely close with each other and interdependent emotionally. They were also negative in outlook and completely lacking in objective viewpoint and sense of responsibility for their actions. If one observed what they thought to be an example of unfair client demand, they would go into a huddle, reinforce each other's negative beliefs and act accordingly. Their negative influence spread far and wide to the other team members, and was noticeable to the client.

Membership of this small group was exclusive: no 'outsiders' were allowed in, even from the greater team. However, their influence was widespread. All attempts to address the situation, to understand the root causes, identify alternative behaviours and lead by example succeeded in influencing some to change. A hard core of two individuals were reluctant to change, to be part of the solution, and after much intervention they had to be removed from the team.

Happily in this example, alternative roles were found elsewhere in the organisation, which, once embraced, brought out the best in their skills, strengths and attitudes. A change in environment and a new culture to which they joined transformed their attitudes and performance. In the absence of the negative influence, the remaining team members rapidly changed and with the addition of new replacement members, the client saw continuous improvements. If this transfer had not been possible, severing employment was the only other alternative.

There are always reasons for dysfunction. Some are understandable, while others are not. Effort to resolve dysfunction brings its reward to all, even when you have to let people go. Knowing your team so you may effectively lead them can prevent the onset of dysfunction.

Suggested learning outcomes and action points

1 Understand the key sources of dysfunction in teams.

2 Consider which sources of dysfunction exist within the individual teams as well as the greater practice team. Examine these in a group meeting; plan this exercise so it cannot be perceived as threatening to the teams.
3 Set a goal of building trust and mastering conflict among team members. Think of how your staff meetings and other communications will look when these have been achieved. Begin with yourself and lead by example.

References

1 Lencioni P. *The Five Dysfunctions of a Team: A Leadership Fable*. San Francisco: Jossey Bass Wiley; 2002.
2 Lencioni P. *Overcoming the Five Dysfunctions of a Team Workbook*. San Francisco: Jossey Bass Wiley; 2005.

Chapter 14

Essential supports for your development

Making your development as a leader and teambuilder easier

Making changes and achieving goals is a whole lot easier when you are working within a supportive environment. This involves consciously designing and managing the elements of your life that have an impact on you. Think of this as though you are putting an extension on top of a building. The first thing you would do is put scaffolding up where the new part is being built. This serves the purpose of supporting the new parts until they are completed. In this analogy you are the building and the scaffolding is your supportive environment.

The scaffolding comprises:

- your physical environment
- your relationships
- the environment in your head (beliefs and attitudes)
- your health
- your personal operating systems
- the workplace culture.

Physical environment

This should inspire, energise or relax you, according to your needs. Consider:

- Do you enjoy calming music during a break or something more energising?
- Do noises easily distract you?
- Does seeing piles of journals or reading material drive you crazy?
- Are there certain clothes that make you feel more efficient, professional or comfortable?
- Are you strongly affected by the temperature of your space or the amount of fresh air you have?
- What impact does your furniture have, especially your chair? Do you think more creatively when you can lean back and put your feet up? Do you think more analytically when you are in an office chair?
- Are you happier when you can walk around and stretch?

Exercise: Optimising your physical environment

Think back over the places you have lived and worked during your life. Which was the best one? What was it about that environment that made it so good?

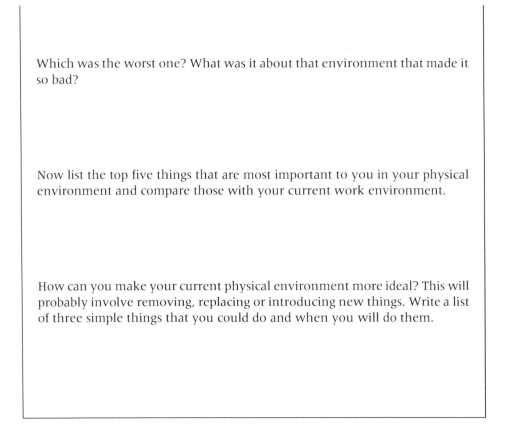

Which was the worst one? What was it about that environment that made it so bad?

Now list the top five things that are most important to you in your physical environment and compare those with your current work environment.

How can you make your current physical environment more ideal? This will probably involve removing, replacing or introducing new things. Write a list of three simple things that you could do and when you will do them.

Your environment to help create change

As a newly qualified physiotherapist I was regularly giving my patients exercises to do and often they weren't being done. I discovered the main reason was not that people couldn't be bothered; it was more a case of them forgetting. Once we introduced prompts in their environment and attached their exercises to part of their routine, like stretching when they were brushing their teeth, a lot more exercise was done.

The same prompts can be used in your environment when you are making changes to your behaviour as a leader and team builder. One of my clients who was starting to use the Covey Time Management Matrix (*see* Chapter 2) had a copy of it pinned above his computer so that whenever he looked up he reinforced his new way of working.

You just need to use your imagination and think of something that works for you.

- A notice on your door saying 'problems welcome when accompanied by solutions' will stop others coming to you with problems only. Your goal is to get them thinking of solutions and to get you out of the habit of taking on the job of 'Mr Fix-It'. Naturally you must first tell your colleagues of this change in approach; the sign is a reinforcement for them and for *you*.

- Closing your door is a good way to tell others you don't want to be disturbed, while an open door is an invitation to enter. Don't expect people to figure this out for themselves: make sure you tell them. A practice manager, whom I coached, decided he needed to close his door, not because he was being disturbed by other people, but because he couldn't help being distracted by the sounds and movement outside.
- If you are in an open-plan environment, having a statue or sign on your desk can be used to signify to others whether you can be disturbed or not. A solid piece of card bent in half with a red traffic light circle on one side and a green one on the other is an easily recognised 'stop/go' sign. Do ensure you use it appropriately.

Your relationships

These may also need reviewing when you are making changes. Relationships span a spectrum from 'drainers' to 'superchargers'. When you have interacted with drainers you may feel like someone has sucked out all your positive energy or dropped a wet blanket over you leaving you feeling miserable. When you have interacted with superchargers you feel lighter, brighter and bursting with energy. When next you interact with people, take note of how you feel before and after to decide what influence they have on you. Aim to invest more time with the superchargers and reduce or eliminate the time spent/wasted with the drainers. Be aware that you fall on this spectrum too and you can choose to be a supercharger yourself.

Sometimes your colleagues or friends don't want you to make positive changes as it will impact the dynamics of the relationship you share. They may feel they have a position of power over you or possess higher self-esteem, while you lack assertiveness or confidence. If you resolve these issues, your 'friend' may lose those feelings that are hurting you but are helping them. If you find that you are moving on but others are trying to hold you back then it's probably time for a heart-to-heart conversation. They may be unenthusiastic about or directly undermining your efforts through actions or words.

Try using the non-violent communication technique or APISWAPED discussed in Chapter 7 (from p. 57) to raise and resolve this issue. Ultimately if they are not going to have a positive influence on you then it's time to seriously consider how you want to interact with them, if at all. If you can't avoid them then be aware of how much time you spend with them and use techniques to protect yourself from their draining affect.

For example, when I was a physiotherapist I had a particular patient who was very insecure and was constantly seeking reassurance. After a few visits, as soon as I saw her, I would start to lose the will to live. This was having a negative impact on my mood and I was concerned it would have a negative impact on our interaction and hence her recovery. The solution for me involved a combination of changing how I communicated with her and a visualisation technique. I imagined putting on a long golden shiny coat which caught each one of her negative comments and questions. I was still bright and sparkling in my gold coat approach while I worked with her and when she left, I pictured myself taking off the coat and throwing it away with all the negativity on it. This worked brilliantly to make me feel a lot less stressed.

The environment in your head

This means your beliefs and attitudes about yourself, other people, the organisation in which you work, in fact everything in your life. These can help or hinder, empower or disempower you. They are therefore essential to consider and to adjust so that they always support you. The exercise 'What are your beliefs?' in Chapter 10 (p. 90) will help you become more aware of your beliefs as well as how to change them.

Sometimes people don't believe that what goes on in their heads has much of an impact on what they do. But, over and over, when people seem unable to take action, or obstacles just keep coming up or nothing seems to be going right for them, it is usually a sabotaging belief creating the problem.

Exercise: How your beliefs affect your behaviour and feelings

Consider this scenario and put yourself in the position of this person.

You have decided that you want to be better at leading your team and you think that your staff meetings are the place to begin. Historically, there tend to be a couple of people who hijack the event and generally moan, stopping you from having the productive meeting you desire.

In the meeting, you are hopeful that you will be able to complete the agenda but as usual one of the staff commences her complaints. You tell her that you need to move on, but she continues her monologue.

Inside, you think: 'She has such a strong personality; I can't compete.' That is your belief. In that position, what do you do next and how do you feel?

Now imagine that you think: 'She has such a strong personality, but I can handle her. This agenda is more important than talking about something we can't change.' That is your belief. In that position what do you do next and how do you feel?

Held back by the first belief, you would most likely have been unable to challenge the person and the meeting would have deteriorated as it had done in the past. Armed with the support of the second belief, which gave you confidence in yourself and a greater purpose to get on with the job, you would probably have seen yourself taking charge of the conversation.

And all of this behaviour derives from your thoughts.

Sometimes your thoughts are not as obvious, particularly your disempowering beliefs.

If you can't actually visualise yourself at the point where your goal has been achieved, then it's unlikely to happen.

You can use this as a test of your beliefs. Can you see yourself challenging difficult behaviour, taking charge of a meeting, inspiring others to adopt a new work process or even going home on time? If you can't, then you probably don't believe it's possible and you begin to sabotage your best intentions.

Exercise: Making new beliefs real

To support the achievement of your goals and creating empowering beliefs, construct in your mind a vivid movie of you at the point where your goal is achieved. For example:

- See yourself confidently handling a complaining staff member during a meeting and achieving the outcome you desire.
- Imagine yourself being assertive at work so that you are on time with your appointments and can leave work at the appropriate time.
- See yourself delegating work to another staff member and feel happy about letting go of control.

In any movie that you create, make sure you can see yourself, the other people and the environmental context, hear what is being said and what you are saying to yourself and step into your shoes and feel your emotions.

Run the movie through your head several times, seeing, hearing and feeling this scenario until it becomes ingrained and easier to re-create in your mind. Continue to run this movie once or twice a day for the next two weeks to help ingrain this belief of what you are able to do. The more you see it happening, the easier it will be for you to do in reality.

Your health

If you are feeling physically fit and healthy you will generally have more energy, be more resilient to stress and have a brighter mood. In my view, your overall health equates to your total energy, which is easy to self-assess because you can literally feel it. A simple equation to illustrate how our energy adds up is:

Total Energy = Energy Boosters minus Energy Drainers

If your drainers are greater than your boosters then you will probably feel tired, lethargic, uninspired or unwell. If they are equal then you will probably be feeling OK but you won't have any reserves to access if you need to.

Your energy boosters and drainers largely consist of the same things:

- food – what and how much you eat
- sleep – quality and how much
- exercise – too much or too little
- relaxation – are you relaxing at all and would you benefit from this?
- emotions – positive or negative
- physical environment – where you live, cluttered or uncluttered, too hot or too cold.

Exercise: Energy booster

Think about each of the above elements to specifically identify what is boosting and draining your energy.

List your energy boosters by considering what makes you feel good or great.

List your energy drainers by considering what you are putting up with.

Looking at your lists, think how you can increase your energy boosters (e.g. listening to energising music more often or reinforcing your boundaries around your free time).

Think of what you can do to eliminate your top energy drainers (e.g. reducing contact with a particular person or hiring someone to do a task that you dislike).

Write an action plan comprising one thing you will do more of and one thing you will do less of.

Your personal operating systems

This means knowing yourself and how you operate best. Some people like to invest 10 minutes each morning to plan their day; otherwise they feel uncomfortable for the rest of the day as though they are not sure what is coming next. Some people know they are best at doing their paperwork first thing in the morning; for others it's easier at the end of the day.

I had a client who hated doing clinics on Friday afternoons. She was tired and couldn't give the patients the care she wanted, nor did she feel she was as sharp with her thinking as at other times during the week. She shuffled her schedule to leave those afternoons for paperwork and was much more efficient in her clinics at other times.

If you know that you work better to a well-structured timetable, then give up trying to be super-flexible. Use a timetable and factor in a block of time during which you are available for others or during which you can catch up on other tasks if you have had unavoidable interruptions. If you have difficulty concentrating for more than an hour reading documents, then schedule lots of breaks or allocate multiple short periods for the task.

The key is to know yourself and work with it; don't fight it. When you try to work in a way that doesn't suit you, the task will always take you much longer and make you less effective.

Exercise: What makes you effective?

Think of a time when you were really efficient in getting all of your work done – all of your 'work' meaning face-to-face clinical jobs, the non-face-to-face clinical tasks, attending meetings, building relationships with colleagues etc.

What habits, routines, structures and support did you have in your personal and professional life that made you more effective? Think big picture. For example, you may have been jogging three times a week, taking planning time each day or having meetings on certain days.

Consider which of these systems, habits or routines could be implemented to help you practise being a better leader and team builder.

Workplace culture

Once you have created a spirit of leadership and teamwork and people feel the benefits and see the good results, the culture of the business can begin to change. This will take a long time, especially if the new culture is a big change. Your business's culture is represented by the norms of behaviour and accepted values among that group of people. The only way these will change is with steady reinforcement and demonstration of the benefits over a substantial period. That's why you can't change a culture first and the behaviours second.

When the culture has been adopted and the staff are actively reinforcing it then the culture itself becomes a support for the development and growth of the organisation. It can be a reference point around which to base decisions and a yardstick against which to measure new recruits. After all, when their values are aligned with the business's values, staff will be happier and more engaged in the workplace.

Remember that the culture of a workplace will need to be flexible according to the environment in which it operates. For example, a doctor who runs their surgery with a culture that 'the patient always comes first' may have been able to manage when the number of patients in the area was smaller. However, if the patient population grows and the doctor is reluctant to take on more staff, they will soon find that adhering to their culture means very late nights, a deteriorating personal life and possibly burnout. The culture (i.e. norms of behaviour) will need to change.

Ask:

- 'What is the culture of this department, team or practice?'
- 'What are the benefits we are getting from this culture and what is it costing us?'

If the benefits don't outweigh the costs, then you should consider whether the culture needs changing and to what.

When you consider these questions, be sure to explore the real culture as demonstrated, not the culture written as part of the mission or vision statement.

I remember going to a general practice for a meeting and while I waited in the reception area I noticed the atmosphere. It was subtle but clear that there was some dissatisfaction among the staff. Quiet murmuring among them and rolling of eyes made it feel like they were preparing for battle. None of this was directed at patients so it appeared there was a battle within the practice. Interestingly, part of the written mission statement of this practice was to develop as a supportive team.

Clearly there was a contrast between what the real culture was and the written culture the management team was aiming for. The reason for the difference in this practice was a toleration of negative, resistant behaviour by some key members of staff which completely disrupted any sense of teamwork. So walk around your department or practice with extra sensitivity to the behaviour and values as demonstrated to get a sense of the culture that is alive.

Suggested learning outcomes and action points

1 Understand the impact of your physical environment, relationships, your beliefs and attitudes, your health and your personal systems on how easily you can make changes.
2 Create an action plan from one of the exercises above: 'What makes you effective?', 'Energy booster' or 'Making new beliefs real'.

Chapter 15

Situations needing extra-strength leadership

In our experience, there are some situations that leaders find particularly challenging:

- handling difficult* behaviour by staff
- handling difficult behaviour by patients towards staff
- times of change such as the retirement, resignation or addition of new staff and moving premises
- leading multidisciplinary teams.

Handling difficult behaviour by staff

A common complaint by staff in the workplace is that 'poor' performers are not dealt with. Remember that performance relates to both the task and the quality of the relationships during task activity. If someone isn't performing, then other staff will often become stressed as they have to take on the resulting extra workload. For example, if a receptionist is rude to a patient and the patient complains, then extra work is created for the practice manager who handles the complaint.

When you as the leader have the opportunity to address poor performance you can send a strong message to all of the staff that you have a fair process. Everybody learns and believes that your primary agenda is to maximise the performance of each individual, the team and the organisation. They also learn that dismissal is the last option but will be used if necessary to uphold the purpose, vision and values of the organisation.

In Chapter 7, 'Leading by compulsion', there are two suggested frameworks for conversations to address difficult behaviour from p. 56. The following framework presumes that you have tried these without success and that the behaviour is not improving. This framework has been based on the process from the article entitled 'How to motivate your problem people' by Nigel Nicholson.[1]

Step 1: Adopt the right attitude

Your attitude, while you gather information before and then during the conversation, needs to be one of curiosity. Your intention should not be to punish the staff member or find an excuse to sack them. Instead of picturing yourself as the judge

---

* This is anything that affects the performance and relationships of the team or of individuals, such as being rude, avoiding being a team player, malicious gossip or performing below agreed standards.

and executioner, picture yourself as a Sherlock Holmes style detective, aiming to get to the bottom of the problem using an objective not a subjective approach.

Begin this process with the positive expectation that once you can show your understanding of the individual you are likely to be able to reach a positive outcome. This will focus your mind on first understanding the other person and second finding a strategy. This is absolutely vital. Without showing your understanding the individual is unlikely to be open and honest. Consequently they will be reluctant to accept or create strategies to solve the existing problems and your suggestions are unlikely to be welcomed or fully committed to.

Also be prepared for the staff member to be unwilling to change their behaviour or performance, despite your best efforts. Bear in mind that revealing the strengths and character of the individual may highlight that their current job or some of their responsibilities are not a good match for them. As already mentioned, if another position is not available or their job cannot be adapted, then the best resolution may be resignation or termination of employment.

Again, remember that your goal is an objective solution, *not* an emotional one. The emotions that temporarily arise from a solution being reached are irrelevant as they do not reflect the solution.

Consider the results and associated emotion in these scenarios:

1 A suitable solution is reached and you are both happy with the outcome.
2 A suitable solution is reached but you feel unhappy because you have had to lead by compulsion, which you are uncomfortable doing. The other person feels unhappy that they will have to change their ways.
3 A weak solution is reached and you both feel happy because you haven't been forced to confront the situation and the other person knows they won't really have to make any changes.
4 No solution is reached and you back down feeling intimidated and the other person is happy they won't have to change.

Step 2: Get the full picture

To do this you must know and understand the person and the events that have led to the need for this conversation. Hopefully, as this person is one of your staff, you will already have some of the answers to the questions below. Talk with the staff member's colleagues, with absolute confidentiality, for background information and discuss the relevant details with the individual during your meeting.

- What are the possible reasons for this person's behaviour or performance?
- Are they having problems in their personal life?
- Do they find their work unfulfilling? Do they feel bored? Do they feel unrecognised?
- Are they struggling with their work volume or the type of work?
- Are they being bullied by another staff member?
- What is really important to them at work?
- What do they need to work well? Is it recognition; is it purpose?
- What is stopping them from working well?

Different perspectives

If there were specific incidents of poor performance/behaviour, review those situations, imagining the event from the individual's perspectives. What might they have been feeling? What might they have been trying to achieve?

Consider the event from the perspective of the person or people interacting with that individual. What might they have been feeling and trying to achieve?

Consider the events from a fly-on-the-wall perspective. What else was contributing to this situation?

Lastly, consider the role that the culture of the workplace and you as the supervisor/manager may have played in the problem. Are you supporting them; are you smothering them; do your communication techniques clash? Is the culture having an impact? Is the staff member afraid of taking risks or admitting mistakes?

Step 3: Prepare for the conversation

Advise the employee one or two days before the event that you need to have a meeting with them to 'review and revise' your working relationship. Reassure them that they don't need to do any preparation and try to meet in a neutral area, so preferably not your office. Also, try to sit perpendicular, rather than opposite each other, as this is less confrontational.

Step 4: The conversation framework: introduction, exploration and solutions.

Introduction

Your **introduction** sets the scene.

Begin by *appreciating* the work and value that the individual brings to the organisation and team.

Objectively explain what the current problem is (usually in terms of behaviour or performance) and the impact of that problem (i.e. effect on their colleagues' behaviour and workload, impact on patient health, the business as a whole).

State your *positive intention* of finding a solution to the problem that works for all parties.

State that the situation cannot continue because of its impact and that it will not be allowed to continue.

Acknowledge that you may not have a full understanding of the situation, including the impact of yourself and other staff, and that you want to explore this in order to find a solution.

Exploration

The **exploration** part of the conversation seeks to find common ground that you can agree on and identify any differences which may or may not be resolvable.

Keep your questions and acknowledgements positive and empathic.

For example: the person says, 'Nobody here cares about the receptionists.' A positive response would be: 'I didn't know you felt that way. Thank you for sharing that. It sounds like you're not getting the recognition or respect you need.' A negative response would be: 'That's not true, you shouldn't feel that way.'

Use the YOW tool to explore what role the individual, other people and the workplace are playing in the problem.

Also *use the questioning technique* known as the *Five Whys* to get the root of a problem. To reduce the chance of making the individual feel defensive ask 'What is the reason for that?' instead of 'Why?'. You may not need to ask the question five times but don't stop before you get to the root of the problem.

For example:

1 Leader: So what was the reason for you raising your voice at Dr Smith?
   Staff member: I was getting angry and frustrated.
2 Leader: And what was the reason for you feeling that way?
   Staff member: I just had so much work on that day and it felt like he was just adding more work for me to do. I really wanted to get home on time for my kids.
3 Leader: And what do you think was the reason for having so much work on that day?
   Staff member: Well, since Sarah left we've all had to pick up her workload so we have a lot extra to do and Dr Smith always leaves it to the last minute to get letters done so we have to drop everything and do them so the patients don't suffer.
4 Leader: OK, so the extra load since Sarah left is taking away the little bit of flexibility that you had in your day. We are in the process of replacing her so that should soon be solved. Meanwhile regarding Dr Smith's letters, what do you think causes him to leave them to the last minute?
   Staff member: He often seems to be running late with his paperwork, but also he's part time so he probably doesn't get the chance to do as much on-site. Maybe that's why all the letters seem to come at once?
5 Leader: Well, until we get a new staff member, this problem may flare up again. I'm sure Dr Smith would be happy to talk about this to find a better way of getting the letters done. Would you be willing to do that?
   Staff member: Yeah, OK.

If the person has trouble being objective or is feeling very emotional, they may need to *release their feelings first* so that they feel understood and heard. You can help them do that by using the non-violent communication technique of empathic listening.

For example:

1 Leader: So what was the reason for you raising your voice at Dr Smith?
   Staff member: We've got so much work to do already and then he comes in telling us we have to get these letters done. We are working our socks off and he just doesn't realise how hard it is.
2 Leader *(empathising with their feelings and needs):* So you were feeling angry and frustrated because you're not being recognised for the hard work you are doing?
   Staff member: Yeah, I just had so much work on that day and it felt like he was adding more for me to do. Besides, I really wanted to get home on time for my kids 'cause I feel like I've been neglecting them lately.
3 Leader *(empathising with their feelings and needs again):* So you were also afraid that you weren't going to be able to have the chance to connect with your kids, which is really important to you.

Staff member *(feeling heard):* Yeah, that's right. When I stay back to get the work done, my family suffers for it.

4   Leader: I'd like to help resolve that situation as this practice does not want the staff or their families to suffer. Would you be willing to look a little more closely at what is happening with your workload so we can see how that might be improved?

Staff member: Yeah, OK.

5   Leader: You mentioned that you had so much work on that day. Was that more work than usual?

Staff member: Well, since Sarah left . . .

Solutions

By the time you reach the **solutions** stage you should both have identified and agreed on some of the elements of the problem as well as know that the needs of the other person have been heard. Now it's time to find solutions.

Review the key sources of the problems that you have explored and check with them: 'Have I got that right?'

Request their input, asking: 'What do you think would be a workable solution?' If that doesn't elicit any response, then ask: 'In an ideal world, what would be a good solution?' What they consider to be impossible may in fact be a realistic option. Alternatively try brainstorming and start by asking what the worst idea would be to fix the problem. As we generate ideas by association, working 'backwards' to a good idea can allow people to be more creative.

Use the YOW tool to explore what role the individual, other people and the workplace can play in the solution.

Suggest your own solutions.

Together, agree on an action plan including what will be done differently, what supports will be put in place to help with doing things differently, what you will measure to know that things have changed, when you will meet to review progress and what the consequences will be if nothing changes.

Affirm with them that you want to keep them and that you want this to work out best for all parties. Don't finish with a threat; finish with sincerity and optimism.

Step 5: Follow-up

At your review meeting, you should have quantitative measurements that tell you what progress has been made as well as qualitative input. If improvements are being made at a satisfactory rate then continue to build on that.

If progress is not being made, explore the reasons for this and then make a decision as to whether the person needs to enter the formal disciplinary process. You may have already covered this in your first meeting when discussing the consequences of not making the required changes.

When people just won't change

Sometimes, despite your very best intentions, people will not recognise or admit that they are part of a problem or accept responsibility for creating the solution. Crunch time for them is often felt when you have stated that the situation must change or when you have commenced the formal disciplinary procedure. At this point, the person may begin to look for another job and leave before you have to terminate their position. This is a resolution to the problem even though it may not be what you hoped for.

You must be careful when terminating someone's position that you adhere to current employment law. It is advisable to seek input from a human resources consultancy or employment lawyers when you create the disciplinary and termination procedures. When you then implement it, *follow it to the letter*.

If you are implementing a major change such as the creation of behavioural standards for the practice, then you must undergo a formal consultation period with your employees. It is advisable to officially state 'this is the start of the consultation period' in writing to your employees and then you must ensure that it is a meaningful consultation. State the current situation, the changes required and the supporting reasons. Ask for their thoughts and feelings and seek to find a solution together. Have as much communication as possible and use a conversation framework similar to the one we have described for individuals. Ultimately, if employees do not agree with the changes, you may need to terminate their position and offer a new job contract, which they may apply for.

Handling difficult behaviour by patients towards staff

'Difficult' behaviour in this scenario amounts to abuse or aggression which has not been provoked. On the one hand you want to keep your staff protected in a positive, supportive work environment, while on the other hand you don't want to alienate your patients or you won't have an income for your business. In our view there is little room for negotiation here. When the staff have not provoked the patient you must support them, even if it means removing a patient from your register.

The most likely scenario is that a patient is very stressed and upset and something minor has 'set them off'. You must investigate and address this behaviour to set an example to the other patients and staff. Invite the patient to discuss this with you in a quiet area and use the non-violent communication technique for the discussion.

For example: 'When you raised your voice and leant toward the receptionist, I felt really distressed because respect and safety are important to me. Would you be willing to discuss what was happening in that situation?'

Allow them time to answer. They may apologise immediately and give you an explanation. In this instance, you can demonstrate your understanding and decide the appropriate action.

'OK, I understand now. I know our receptionist is quite upset though. Would you be willing to explain this to her so she can appreciate your position?'

Alternatively they may point out things about the practice that irritate them. They may have some valid points to make, so be empathic and acknowledge their feelings and needs:

> So you were angry that there was a delay in seeing the doctor because your health is very important. Giving you excellent healthcare is very important to us too, so we are looking into what went wrong. Once we know what happened I can advise you of what we are doing to prevent

it happening again. I'd also like your input if you have any solutions to suggest. Is that acceptable to you?

If they do not have a valid point (e.g. complaining about not being given an emergency appointment so they can attend outside of work hours) your conversation will be different:

> So you were angry that you were not given an emergency appointment. I appreciate that you have difficulty arranging appointments around your work hours. However, the availability of the emergency appointments is subject to very strict medical criteria in order to preserve that time for people who are very, very unwell. In your situation, we recommend that you take one of the earliest or latest appointments to minimise the disruption to your work. Alternatively you could use a drop-in clinic or you may need to take sick leave.

Another scenario is that you are faced with a person being abusive because that is the way in which they choose to communicate. Decide how many warnings you wish to give before removing them from your register and make sure that you do this in conjunction with a formal policy. Your policy, which must be known by patients, should describe what behaviour from them is acceptable and unacceptable.

This is sometimes defined under patient responsibilities in the practice leaflet or notices in the waiting area. I would suggest that, when new patients register with the practice, they are given an agreement form documenting the practice's and the patient's responsibilities and seek an agreement from the patient at the time. As stated earlier, you are then able to hold people accountable to an agreed standard rather than it appearing to be a personal attack. Your conversation or letter of notice then involves stating the responsibilities they had agreed to or your policy on aggression, the violations of those standards and the consequences.

The final scenario is that people are abusive due to a mental illness. This is not common in my experience; however, it has happened and should be prepared for. The only different factor in this scenario is that it may be more difficult to reason with the person.

Simple safety procedures involve ensuring that you are not alone with the individual. It is valuable to know those in the practice's patient population who may be at risk of having an acute mental health episode.

Even if the person is angry and agitated you may be able to reason with them, using the rapport-building techniques described earlier. However, if they are having a psychotic episode they may not believe or even be hearing you. Some simple advice to remember is don't rush them and do give them your full attention. Don't presume and suggest how they are feeling. Instead, ask them: 'Are you feeling afraid/angry/upset?' Ask them how you can help them and explain what you can and can't do for them. Don't stand or sit too close to them; be to the side of them not directly opposite and give them the same amount of eye contact that they are giving you.

If they are paranoid they may be worried about others conspiring against them so give them less rationale for these thoughts by removing dictaphones and attending to them, not the computer. The fewer distractions, the better.

Always have a procedure specific to this scenario which if possible will involve identifying the individual and contacting their psychiatrist or social worker. It may be necessary to involve the police as they have the power to restrain someone against their will. Note that you may need to let them leave before contacting the police if they are a threat to themselves or others.

It is important to have a 'handling difficult behaviour' policy created in conjunction with all staff. This should document the order of who to contact should the initial staff member be unable to manage the situation and if the situation deteriorates (i.e. the team leader, practice manager, another management team member and the police).

Ensure that staff are comfortable with the suggested dialogue and they feel sufficiently assertive to use it. Knowing that they are 'allowed' to walk away from aggressive patients or to ask them to come back 'when they are prepared to discuss the issue more constructively' often gives the staff the support they need from management.

Also always consider the environment. For example, in the treatment rooms/offices, set up the doctor's/nurse's desk closer to the door than the patient's chair. Could someone jump over the reception desk and is there room for the receptionist to move out of harm's way? As always, the staff member involved will be able to give you valuable information.

Times of change

Another common complaint in general practices is that there is too much change. 'Why can't we get used to one thing, before they introduce another?' Unfortunately the only constant feature in healthcare is change.

The problem with any change is that even if it is for the better in the medium or long term, there is always short-term upheaval, a sense of uncertainty and consequent stress. If you look at any list of sources of stress, it is all to do with change; even getting married or buying your dream house. The way people respond to change affects how effective they are in supporting the change process and their stress levels. For some it is a challenge and a learning experience. For others it is a nuisance that they will complain about and resist.

General practices are subjected to a lot of changes from outside such as the government and General Medical Council, but they also create their own changes from within such as moving premises, acquiring another practice or the resignation, retirement or addition of key staff members, particularly in the management team.

Having a framework to follow for any change increases the likelihood of a smooth journey to a successful result. With this in mind, we recommend applying the approach described in John P Kotter's book *Leading Change*.[2] His process is based on work with large organisations so we have described it here in the context of smaller businesses:

- Stage 1: Establishing a sense of urgency.
- Stage 2: Creating the guiding coalition.
- Stage 3: Developing a vision and strategy.
- Stage 4: Communicating the change vision.

- Stage 5: Empowering broad-based action.
- Stage 6: Generating short-term wins.
- Stage 7: Consolidating gains and producing more change.
- Stage 8: Anchoring new approaches in the culture.

Stage 1: Establishing a sense of urgency

Complacency is a dangerous state to have in any business, especially healthcare. Complacency related to patient care can literally be deadly. In relation to business operations it can mean missing opportunities for increasing income and improving healthcare or putting up with ineffective processes which make for a more stressful work environment. Inundated with external demands, many practices have a sense that they couldn't be bothered or don't have time to make improvements.

If you find yourself talking in 'buts' – for example, 'That team don't get on very well but . . .' or 'We should do something about that but . . .' or 'That really could be a lot better but . . .' – then you are in the complacency trap. The problems that you are describing are just not 'painful' enough for you to do anything about it.

One particular practice that I worked with was quite different. It didn't have any significant problems; however, they knew that the partner that did most of the 'running the business' work was retiring in a few years. Rather than panicking three years later and then figuring out what running the business entailed, they were planning and gradually making changes well in advance. In reality it would probably take them a year or two to make the changes that would ensure the continued smooth running of the business when the retirement occurred.

There are several things that can reduce complacency and create the sense of urgency that is necessary to create action.

- Take a mental walk into the future (three months, one year, three years and five years) and see what will happen if the problem is not resolved. Consider the cost in terms of the staff's mental and physical health, patient care, income for the practice, ease of staff recruitment, staff turnover. If you have staff who 'don't get it', hold a meeting and ask them to do the same exercise.
- Give a reality check to staff and present objective findings such as patient dissatisfaction, low performance outcomes or a list of errors that have occurred. If a single team is struggling, first do this with them alone and explore the reasons for the problems. If they report a negative influence from other staff/ teams or request involvement from other staff as part of their solution, then a combined meeting is required.
- Get an external facilitator for a truly open conversation between staff to air grievances. Seeing issues and problems spelt out on a flipchart is a good way to make them more real for everyone.

Stage 2: Creating the guiding coalition

Those that make up the 'guiding coalition' are the decision makers and drivers of change. Not everyone in the management team has to be involved, especially if it is a large team. However, all members of management must be committed to the decisions made. If anyone in a position of leadership demonstrates resistance or complacency they will quash other staff members' enthusiasm and give permission for staff to behave in the same way. This is leadership by example in the worst way.

A practice manager once told me how they were struggling with a restructuring project when one of the receptionists was promoted to team leader. The problem they faced was that the new team leader still felt that she was one of the receptionists and that team had previously portrayed an 'us and them' feeling toward the management team. Consequently, suggestions and plans from management were being undermined by the team leader when she communicated them to the staff.

In this case, it was vital that the team leader associate her role within the practice as part of the management team, not the receptionists. Having her participate in management meetings so she could see the big picture of what the practice was striving to achieve and giving her training in people management and leadership would have helped shift how she identified herself within the practice.

When choosing who will make up the coalition, look for skills of management and leadership. Remember that doesn't mean they have to hold a formal position as a manager. Also, beware of people who may be very capable but have large egos and dominate all of the proceedings.

Once the members have been selected, it is vital that they have a strong team relationship. This may not be the case if the team leaders don't often work together so investing in protected time for teambuilding exercises will be very worthwhile. Remember that the fundamental ingredient for a strong team is trust. This is not easy to develop through occasional daily interactions, which are very different to sharing and critiquing ideas and strategies. Trust needs to be built in this context.

Stage 3: Developing a vision and strategy

Having a vision is like having a compass for the practice. It will guide and simplify every decision as you ask: 'Will this action/behaviour support our vision?' Even when the action may involve short-term pain, if the answer to this question is 'yes' then the long-term gain becomes the focus. The 'change' vision may be very different to the existing vision of the business.

For example, change visions may include:

- 'We are going to provide the highest level of healthcare in the county.'
- 'We are going to make how we operate as a team as important as our patient care.'

Stage 4: Communicating the change vision

People don't remember things after hearing them once and if the management team has a poor history of following things through, what you say may not even be believed. The key is to communicate the vision as often as possible, informally and formally. Whenever a decision is being made, state the vision and then evaluate the decision in relation to that. At the end of a meeting, ask: 'What have you done this week that has supported the vision?' Have the statement framed and erected where it will be seen often. Ask people what they think about the vision; is it clear and believable? Most importantly, ensure that the management team and guiding coalition are behaving according to the vision and that they hold others account-able to the same standards.

Stage 5: Empowering broad-based action

Everyone must be part of change to make it successful. Seeking and accepting input from everyone, from the cleaner to the partners, and giving them responsibilities, will encourage broad-based action. If staff identify developmental needs to support them with the change process then efforts should be made to meet them. Problems may also be found in processes that do not support the change you are trying to implement. For example, you may want to enhance relationships within your team but there is no time for meetings.

Often practices have staff that they do not employ but still provide a service on behalf of the practice such as health visitors and physiotherapists. For any goal that affects the practice, invite them to contribute their ideas and be responsible for supporting the change.

Stage 6: Generating short-term wins

Most of the changes we have mentioned take several months, if not years, to fully implement. If you wait until that time to offer rewards, morale will probably be very low. Imagine teaching a child to walk. If you waited until they walked 10 steps in a row before giving any praise or encouragement, they would probably never get there. The encouragement that you give them after they manage to stand up motivates them to keep going.

When you are setting out the steps that must occur to achieve the change, allow for a reward to be given at each point. Ensure that you have an objective result which you are celebrating such as the completion of a flowchart for a new triage clinic, or the creation of a job description for a new partner.

This may be a 'thank you' or 'well done' lunch for everyone, which recognises their hard work. Immediate recognition for any particularly challenging tasks also keeps momentum and morale high. Even if the change only affects the partnership – for example, restructuring responsibilities – take the time as a partnership to reward yourselves and the practice manager who will no doubt be involved.

Seeing these short-term successful results can also help to persuade others, who have been resistant to the change, to be more supportive.

Stage 7: Consolidating gains and producing more change

The lesson for general practices in this stage is to maintain urgency and resist complacency and the tendency to 'relax' progress. With changes such as moving or the retirement of a partner, the final result will most likely occur no matter what. However, if progress hasn't been maintained, there will be last-minute panic and disorder which could have been prevented.

'Producing more change' is not essential. However, to fully utilise the work that has been done to date, it is valuable to review lessons learned with all staff and consider how they can be applied to other areas of the business. Once people have been through significant change they can see the direct and indirect improvements that result. For example, creating a greater share of management responsibilities among members of a partnership has the direct result of reducing the workload on one or two members and increasing the workload on the others. Indirect results are likely to be that the other partners discover they have more talents than they realised; their new responsibilities bring them into more frequent contact with other staff, allowing relationships to develop; and, as they review the processes associated with their new responsibility, they find ways to be more efficient.

Stage 8: Anchoring new approaches in the culture

This step is particularly relevant when you are making changes in attitudes and behaviour within your organisation. This usually occurs in conjunction with a more tangible change such as acquiring another practice or improving results from a particular team.

The definition given by Kotter is that:

> *Culture* refers to norms of behavior and shared values among a group of people. *Norms of behavior* are common or pervasive ways of acting that are found in a group and that persist because group members tend to behave in ways that teach these practices to new members, rewarding those who fit in and sanctioning those who do not. *Shared values* are important concerns and goals shared by most of the people in a group that tend to shape group behaviour and that often persist over time even when group membership changes.[2]

One of the most easily recognised cultures which has existed in medical training is 'if you can't take the heat, get out of the kitchen'. This has never been spelt out for new recruits but has resulted in doctors stoically struggling on with difficult people or circumstances and considering it unacceptable to seek help. Fortunately this culture has recently begun to change, though very slowly.

Multiple groups or teams may also have their own culture. A practice I mentioned earlier had a nursing team that did not actively involve new staff members, which created a culture of 'old and included' and 'new and excluded'. The practice's management team however had a culture of 'everyone involved'.

The difficulty with challenging a culture is that it is usually not written down or consciously decided. Objective observation is the only way to identify the behaviours creating the culture, followed by attempting to understand what is driving such behaviour.

Changing behaviour and hence culture can be extremely difficult as we have already discussed.

Success is more likely when the following occur simultaneously:

- The management team leads by example, demonstrating the desired new behaviours.
- The new culture is reinforced and discussed at every opportunity.
- New staff are evaluated with the new culture in mind.
- Staff that do not fit or agree with the new culture are allowed to leave.

- Reasons for resistance to change are explored and obstacles are identified and overcome.
- The good results that occur from the new culture are highlighted.

A final warning from Kotter is that trying to change a culture on its own is virtually impossible. It tends to be achieved only after new behaviour produces benefits for a sustained period and people associate that the results have arisen from the change.

Leading multidisciplinary teams

Multidisciplinary teams bring a particular set of leadership challenges namely:

- staff with different levels of education and methods of learning
- different levels of commitment and engagement between those with a financial investment in the practice, employees and those who work with the practice but are employed by another organisation
- the possibility of staff having negative attitudes related to pay, roles or responsibilities.

What to do about these challenges

1 When running meetings, training or teambuilding activities you must be flexible with your communication and presentation style. Once your information has been presented, then ascertain whether people have actually understood it. When bringing doctors with over six years of university study and administration staff with significantly fewer years of study together, there may be reluctance on behalf of both parties to speak up if they don't understand. The doctors 'should' know it all and the admin staff don't want to look like they don't know. In this situation it is vital that the people seen to be in the more senior role lead by example. Even if they do understand a concept, they can encourage others to speak up by saying, 'Can you give an example so I'm sure I understand?' or asking for further clarification.

2 Gaining greater commitment and engagement from staff, whether they are employed by you or not, will have a positive impact on the entire workplace. Making the practice vision commonly known means people focus on what they do and why they do it, not who they work for. Seeking and valuing everyone's input regarding improvements and feedback on the practice will always give people a stronger sense of involvement. This is particularly important for those who believe they have valuable contributions to make. If they do not have that opportunity, then they will inevitably feel some dissatisfaction.

For those staff that work with you but not for you, it is important that you develop a positive relationship with them and their employer. Understand the terms under which they work and the scope that exists for them to participate more fully in the practice operations. When I worked in a general practice as a physiotherapist I was told I could attend staff meetings 'if I want[ed] to', indicating that there was no real desire from the practice owners for me to attend. I'd also been told that if I have any ideas on how to improve a process then share them, but without a clear process on how to do that it was awkward to chase the manager to have such conversations.

3   When staff air their negative attitudes regarding pay, roles or responsibilities it often comes across as 'I could do your job, you're nothing special' or 'You shouldn't be paid more than me, my job's just as important'. This can either be irritating or become dangerous if the person performs a task they are not legally qualified to do. To address this situation, have a serious conversation with the person about their attitude. Using the non-violent communication method you could say: 'When you make the comment that you could do my job, I feel angry because I have a need for respect for the hard work and years of study that I have invested to get this job. Would you be willing to stop making comments like that?' You can also refer to the roles and responsibilities set out in their job description and the behavioural standards that you may have for your practice staff.

   If they persist with implying that they could do your job, repeat the request from the above dialogue and preface it with 'You're probably right; however, for now, we have distinct roles and responsibilities to adhere. Would you be willing to stop making comments like that?'

If you have teams on separate geographical sites it is important for the teams to feel part of the one practice. To achieve this, there needs to be as many connections between them as possible such as:

- utilising technology to support close communication such as web-cams and conference calls
- representatives from the admin, medical and nursing teams that meet to discuss progress and challenges
- staff meetings where *everyone* meets except for a skeleton shift left in the practices; there needs to be a roster for this so everyone gets to participate
- teambuilding activities on away days to deepen relationships
- sharing of successes and lessons learned between practices.

Ultimately, more effort is required to bring multiple disciplines together; however, the richness of that diversity makes it worthwhile.

Suggested learning outcomes and action points

1   Learn the steps to handling difficult behaviour by staff.
2   Review the framework for handling difficult behaviour by staff and identify what you already do and what you want to do more of.
3   Find a local trainer in non-violent communication at www.cnvc.org and complete the foundation course.
4   Review the last significant change that was implemented in relation to the process described and identify what you would do differently.
5   Discuss with the teams how strongly they feel part of the bigger picture of the practice. Seek their suggestions on how to make that sense of team stronger.

References

1 Nicholson N. How to motivate your problem people. *Harvard Business Review.* January 2003; **81**: 57–65.
2 Kotter JP. *Leading Change.* Boston: Harvard Business School Press; 1996.

Further reading

• Johnson S. *Who Moved My Cheese? An Amazing Way to Deal with Change in Your Work and in Your Life.* London: Vermillion; 1999.

Index